PYRAMID ON THE PRAIRIE

CRAIG MINER

Pyramid On The Prairie

Copyright © 2011 Riordan Clinic

No part of this book may be reproduced or transmitted in any form or by any means electronic or mechanical, including photocopying or by any information storage without permission in writing from the copyright owner.

Photos by Steve Harper

Cover design, book design and layout by Jim L. Friesen

Library of Congress Control Number: 2012933553

International Standard Book Number: 978-0-9850681-0-3

Printed in the United States of America by Mennonite Press, Inc., Newton, KS, www.mennonitepress.com

DEDICATION

Published in honor of my husband, Dr. Hugh D. Riordan, a maverick and charismatic physician, and Olive W. Garvey, a bold and visionary philanthropist. Hugh and Olive conceived of The Center for the Improvement of Human Functioning, which became well known and highly regarded for its patient-centered nutritional approach to healing.

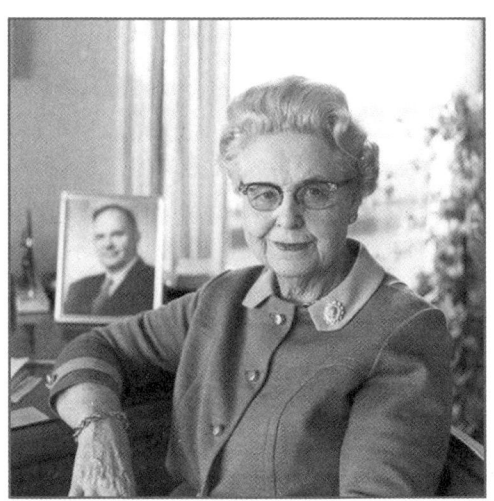

OLIVE W. GARVEY
Businesswoman and philanthropist.

FOREWORD

Anyone who has driven along the northern edge of Wichita, Kansas, has likely been struck by the sight of seven geodesic domes and a white pyramid rising from the prairie. This collection of unusual buildings is home to an alternative health center established by two remarkable people: Hugh D. Riordan and Olive W. Garvey.

My husband, Hugh, was a physician ahead of his time; Olive was a generous philanthropist who understood the value of his foresight. In 1975, he and Olive conceived of The Center for the Improvement of Human Functioning. Today, it is well known and highly regarded for its patient-centered, nutritional approach to healing.

About a decade ago, Hugh commissioned Dr. Craig Miner, the Willard W. Garvey Distinguished Professor of Business History and former chair of the history department at Wichita State University, to undertake the writing of a history of The Center. At the conclusion of Dr. Miner's efforts, however, Hugh was reticent to have it published. Hugh died in 2005 and the manuscript lay idle for five years, until it turned up recently while I was going through Hugh's extensive personal papers.

Although I was very familiar with The Center's many programs and services in the areas of wellness, nutrition, and vitamin/mineral research, I had little to do with its operation. I had been busy raising a large family of six children, practicing my profession as a Registered Nurse, pursuing advanced degrees in my chosen field, and working as a Professor of Nursing at Wichita State University.

I found Miner's manuscript fascinating and I learned a lot from it. The story reflects the tumultuous changes in health care over the course of the last quarter of the 20th century. The book gives the reader a glimpse into the struggles of doctors of the time who sought to incorporate "holistic" care in their practices while experimenting with new nutritional approaches to treatment.

In reading the Miner manuscript, I came to a different conclusion than did Hugh: I felt that Dr. Miner, whom *The Wichita Eagle* called "Kansas' premier historian" upon his death in 2010, had created a revealing, historically significant, and accurate document that I believed deserved to be disseminated.

I decided to discuss the possibility and advantages of going forward with publication with Susan Miner, Craig's widow. I also consulted with members of The Center's Board and some key staff members. All agreed that the story needed to be published. And so, here it is.

Jan Riordan

CONTENTS

Chapter 1 The Doctor And The Lady...........1

Chapter 2 Throwing a Rope.......................29

Chapter 3 Personal Health Control............65

Chapter 4 One of a Kind 95

Chapter 5 The Master Facility..................133

Chapter 6 Health Hunters 161

Chapter 7 A New Era...............................203

Epilogue..229

Favorite Sayings of Hugh 233

Journal Articles 235

About the Author....................................249

Chapter One
The Doctor and the Lady

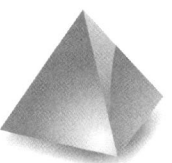

In May 1975, Dr. Hugh Desaix Riordan, Dr. Carl Pfeiffer, and Dr. Bill Schul were welcomed into a pleasant and spacious corner office on the top floor of the Ray Hugh Garvey office building in Wichita, Kansas. It was the headquarters of Garvey, Inc. and the Garvey Foundation. The former concern had until recently operated a substantial and diversified business empire, including, among many other interests, a major independent petroleum exploration and development corporation, a group of grain elevators with around a quarter billion bushels of storage capacity, holdings of over 100,000 acres of farmland, a gasoline retailing company, and 2,000 rental housing units in Wichita. Those companies had been spun off to the next generation of the Garvey family, but the two-building office complex remained along with enough other business to be the envy of most operators. The second entity for which decisions were made in that corner office, the Garvey Foundation, was, and had been for 15 years, one of the major philanthropic forces in the state of Kansas. Among its many achievements were substantial support of Friends University in Wichita and Washburn University in Topeka, the establishment of public television stations in both Wichita and Topeka, and making an enormous difference in the sweep and quality of the local and regional YMCA.

PYRAMID ON THE PRAIRIE

But it was hardly an ordinary executive suite. For one thing, it was decorated much like a home, with a sofa, a credenza, paintings, and memorabilia from world travel. For another, the person behind the desk, the one in charge of all this, was not only a woman, but a grandmother and great grandmother, eighty-one years old. Olive White Garvey had taken over the Garvey family enterprises in 1959 when her husband, entrepreneur Ray Garvey, was killed in an auto accident, and both the business and the philanthropies had not only survived but grown and prospered vigorously since. The three doctors knew that Mrs. Garvey had wide-ranging interests and was a considerable reader as well as a published writer of fiction, non-fiction and plays. And they knew that among her interests were medicine and nutrition, although the depth and extent of that interest was doubtless not guessed at by any of them. A favorite Biblical quote of hers was from *Proverbs*: "with all thy getting, get understanding."[1]

Mrs. Garvey had read *Nutrition and Your Mind* by George Watson, which she had begun one day with enthusiasm while under the hairdryer. She had also read the publications of Pfeiffer, who was working in Princeton, New Jersey, and the work of Dr. Roger Williams on nutrition and on the importance of understanding the unique biochemistry of individuals. She had gone to grade school with Karl Menninger,

---

[1] There are a number of published sources for the life of Olive White Garvey. She herself wrote (with Virgil Quinlisk) a biography of her husband, entitled *The Obstacle Race: The Story of Ray Hugh Garvey* (San Antonio: The Naylor Company, 1970), which included much about herself, and a volume called *Once Upon a Family Tree* (1980), which was a personal account of her life and ancestry. In addition there is Billy Mack Jones, *Olive White Garvey: Humanitarian, Corporate Executive, Uncommon Citizen* (Wichita: Center for Entrepreneurship, 1985) and Craig Miner's *Garvey, Inc.: Expectations to Equity* (Wichita: privately printed, 1992) which documents her role in Garvey, Inc. after 1959. She kept scrapbooks, which were a source for these paragraphs also, as were the author's many talks with her, some of them videotaped. I knew "OWG" well, our acquaintance beginning in the 1950s through my family, but always from afar until 1985, when I began working for her son Willard and we met regularly at her corner office in the Garvey building to talk about her still long list of ideas and enterprises. After her death I designed an exhibit about her. I have drawn on all this here.

founder of the famous Kansas psychiatric clinic, and had dared to discuss with that master the shortcomings of Freudian theories and the frustrations of therapy along those lines. Her practical Quaker background and her no nonsense experience as a mother and a businesswoman had led her to question whether it was always necessary to delve into childhood experience or sexual practice to explain or treat a spiritual malaise that might as well be traced to a sugar imbalance or a B vitamin deficiency.[2] "I always felt," she wrote, "that psychiatry was an inexact science.... For years, one of my inner irritants has been popular, permissive, irresponsible psychology, which the general public has embraced as gospel and which has all but destroyed our society. And when I learned that Freud, the father of much of this thought, had based his dictum that all motivation is based on sex on observation of caged animals in the zoo where there was scant opportunity for any other type of activity, it strengthened my prejudices." Mrs. Garvey had recently tried to give money to several regional universities for nutritional research and had been turned down.[3]

Dr. Schul, author of many books and articles, was doing a six-month study for the Garvey Foundation on the holistic approach to the multiple origins of disease. "While this involvement [of the foundation]," he wrote in March 1974, "may include financial support to research and clinical facilities, the immediate task is to continue the study of research findings and to pull this material together in a manner that it can serve as a useful guide to both professional and lay persons seeking additional sources of information. It will also serve to provide direction for the Board of Directors of the Garvey Foundation."[4] Schul visited Roger Williams in Austin, Texas, early in April 1974. Williams confessed to a colleague a few days later that he had no idea of the resources of the

---

2 See note 1.
3 *Lake Region Echo* (Alexandria, MN), Aug. 10, 1983, clip in History Scrapbook #2, CIHF Archives, Wichita, Kansas. Angelia Herrin, "Trying to Go Beyond," *Wichita Eagle Beacon*, Sept. 5, 1982, History Scrapbook #1, CIHF Archives.
4 Letter, Bill D. Schul to Roger J. Williams, March 11, 1974, Clayton Institute Archives, Austin, Texas. Thanks to Dr. Don Davis for providing photocopies of the Schul/Williams correspondence.

Garvey family, and so suggested that maybe the Foundation might fund the distribution to young doctors of copies of *Physician's Handbook of Nutrition*. That, at least, would sow a small seed. He had learned since that the family resources amounted to $240 million and that "they are definitely interested in health, nutrition and preventative medicine."[5]

It was Schul who suggested to his two associates that they might like to meet Cliff Allison, who was the chief operating officer of the Garvey Foundation, and this led to a ten-minute meeting with Mrs. Garvey.[6] Surely, the combination of doctors was no accident. Pfeiffer was studying the effects of nutritional changes on mental illness, and Riordan, while he was a practicing psychiatrist without deep background in nutrition or laboratory research, was as close as could be found to someone who might be temperamentally, philosophically, entrepreneurially, and professionally qualified to advance holistic medicine in Wichita. He had six children and was married to a nurse-educator. He had experience in political campaigns involved in selling ideas. He had been special consultant to the executive vice-president of the American Medical Association, the first time a physician had filled that post. He had been rehired in that post six different times, after being fired five different times, each time for his criticisms of the organization, which eventually were accepted as accurate.[7] He was an experienced speech-writer and public speaker. His companies, Psyche, Inc. and Four Thirty Four Group (located at 434 N. Oliver), were consulting nationally with companies and school systems in communications, audio-visual production, and motivational training for their employees. From that,

---

5 Letter, Williams to Dr. Francis Woidich, April 4, 1974, ibid. A 1983 article estimated the Garvey family controlled a business empire worth $500 million. They were one of the nation's richest families, ranking with the Fords and Kennedys in wealth if not in publicity. Amazingly, they were only the second wealthiest family in Wichita. The Kochs, who were even more private, topped them. *Wichita Eagle Beacon*, June 26, 1983, in History Scrapbook #1(a), CIHF Archives.
6 The account of the initial meeting with Olive Garvey and Hugh Riordan's background for it is, unless otherwise noted, derived from Interviews, Dr. Hugh Riordan with Craig Miner, May 20, 27, 1998, and Audiotape of talk by Hugh Riordan, May 1, 1997.
7 Interview, Dr. Hugh Riordan with Craig Miner, October 22, 1998.

his work with Pfeiffer on mental illness, and his practice of orthomolecular medicine in his partnership with Dr. Fowler Poling in Wichita, he well recognized the role of health and nutrition in the complex mix that constitutes good health.[8] But the doctors had no inkling just how fortuitous the timing and accidents of this meeting would turn out to be, nor how substantial its long-term results.

The meeting went well. Mrs. Garvey gave each of the physicians a copy of one of her books. Riordan's was a tome on political philosophy with the blunt title *Produce or Starve*. It was abundantly clear that, however kindly this nice old woman might seem, she was hardly a mellifluous ninny. But Riordan was nonplussed when in the midst of their polite chat Pfeiffer blurted out to Garvey that she really ought to give Riordan money to establish a lab in Wichita to study the effects of nutrition. So unprepared was Riordan for such a question that when he got a request later from Allison to submit a proposal, he had to call Pfeiffer to ask him just what kind of a lab it was that he wished to establish. Nor was he sanguine about the chances of funding. One of his pieces of information about Olive Garvey, taken from her book, was that she did not trust in businessmen with beards; Riordan had a beard.

There were questions too about why he should make a proposal at all. Such an opportunity would require him to give up a successful mix of psychiatric practice and consulting in motivation and audio-visual applications. Also, in establishing a nutrition lab to treat mental illness he would be pursuing a field that was so controversial in medical circles that it was often unremorsefully referred to as quackery. He was accustomed to being regarded as a maverick, but such a project could and probably would lead to criticism from colleagues that bordered on abuse.

It was not, however, Riordan's nature to be swayed much by such considerations. He had developed a firm sense of security about himself early in life, along with an awareness that strongly defended but absurd views and behavior even among the well-educated were not only pos-

---

8 Some of the newsletters produced by that group in 1974 are included in History Scrapbooks, vol. 1, CIHF Archives. See also "The Humanistic Shrink," *The Wichitan* (Dec, 1978) in History Scrapbook #1, CIHF Archives.

sible, but to be expected. His response to that insight was not satire or resignation, but disciplined, focused, and pragmatic action. If not necessarily a revolutionary, he had the character at least of a reformer.

Several powerful experiences in his own life had reinforced that combination of healthy skepticism and determined action in him. As a child he had observed his brother cured of a streptococcal throat infection, which made him delirious for 30 days and led the attending doctors to predict his early demise. Riordan's father, however, had read an article in *Time* magazine about the discovery of sulfa drugs. His father was an economics professor at Marquette University, not a physician. However, he could read and think, and the doctors treating his son fortunately would and did listen to what he had to say. They had never heard of sulfa. It was not even in use in the US yet and had to be ordered from Germany. But he ordered some. When it came, they stirred the yellow powder into tomato juice and gave it to the boy. Within 72 hours he was no longer delirious and in two weeks he was entirely well.

The miracle was partly the sulfa, but partly the parent's willingness to buck the local establishment and use his own head. Later Riordan learned that sulfa drugs had been discovered fourteen years before the episode with the yellow powder and the tomato juice, so that "the entire course of my brother's illness was unnecessary." And that was par for the course. A study of medical history revealed to him that the usual time delay in medicine from discovery to implementation was something on the order of forty years.

A second set of epiphanous experiences came when Riordan was in medical school at the University of Wisconsin. Once he got a severe strep throat. The doctor to whom he went gave him two choices. He could take the latest antibiotic, aureomycin, or he could take Vitamin C. The drug would cure him in three days and cost $7; the C would take six days and cost fifty cents. The impecunious medical student took the C and was well in a week. It was a characteristic of the man that no lesson of anything that ever happened to him was lost.

Another discovery came when his class performed a nutrition test with rats. Each group of students had six rats, which were fed a perfect diet except for one nutrient. In each case the missing nutrient was different (with Riordan's group it was folic acid), but in all cases the result was the same: the rats became very ill. They became sicker and sicker and eventually staggered when they walked. When the nutrient was restored, so was their health. Riordan found that experiment "very impressive," and so did his 75 classmates. Many remembered it vividly when Riordan surveyed them many years later. But they did not correlate and apply the lesson as it related to the care of people. Only one besides Riordan had in his later career done anything significant with nutrition except in cases of anemia and other obvious nutritional problems.

As he specialized in the treatment of mental illness, the subject of nutrition continued to come to the fore in the young psychiatrist's experience. When he worked at the Wisconsin Diagnostic Center he tested people with psychological problems for porphyria, a metabolic disorder found to cause certain of these diseases. Again the nutrition connection was there.

Riordan's arrival in Wichita in 1957 had been the result of the same kind of independent study, observation, and consequent action that marked his other decisions. Ignoring all the vague advice about the "prestigious" places to go for internships and residencies, he and two other medical students sent questionnaires all over the country. Almost none of the replies from hospital administrators answered any of their specific questions. They simply sent brochures and a standard packet. Wichita was different. Richard Stone, the administrator of St. Francis, the largest private hospital west of the Mississippi, answered every question in detail and in addition explained to them why Wichita was such a great place to live. All three of them came.

Nutrition again entered into his work. Riordan, soon going into practice with Dr. Fowler Poling, learned that intravenous doses of vitamin B could keep some people out of the state mental hospital. A Boston flight surgeon who had been successful helping airline pilots told Riordan, himself a considerable pilot, that intravenous vitamin B was also a way to prevent time zone fatigue. Poling was a true mentor to Riordan, leading him often into new modes of thought. When

Poling later died in an automobile accident, it caused reflections in Riordan too about the importance of doing what one loved while tenuous life lasted.

Riordan met Dr. Pfeiffer at a lecture in Vancouver. He had taken one look at Riordan at that time and said, "You must have had a really rough time three months ago." In fact, that was when Riordan had had his first attack of gout. Pfeiffer noticed a large white spot on Riordan's thumbnail, a sign of zinc deficiency. Riordan had had white spots on his nails as a child. Once a doctor had told his mother it was because he had bad thoughts, and Riordan had known he was right, so did not look for another explanation.

Pfeiffer's observation was a revelation that not only helped Riordan personally, but, Pfeiffer thought, applied to about 20% of schizophrenias. When fingernail spots and knee joint pain were combined, this dread mental illness could be relieved by supplementation with zinc and vitamin B6. The only problem was that neither the patients nor their relatives would believe it could be so simple. They would abandon the vitamins time and time again, sink back into their madness and only slowly recognize that in fact nutrition was the key. "We always like to see somebody who is crazy and who has knee-joint pain and white spots on their fingernails," Riordan said years later. "They're going to be fixed up in a hurry."

In those years of Wichita psychiatric practice, Riordan had also met Linus Pauling at a conference on the West coast. Pauling was a Nobel prizewinner, but that did not protect him from contemptuous comments concerning his theories on the usefulness of vitamin C. How did he weather all those attacks from doctors, Riordan asked him. The answer was memorable: "Hugh," Pauling said, "you have to understand if your colleagues aren't up on something they tend to be down on it."

So there he was: the independent character, the careful observer, constantly getting the message time and again, here and there, that the simple expedient of studying and regulating what one put into one's body was a powerful tool in maintaining wellness and in treating chronic disease. And here was Garvey, a philanthropist who was an individualist of the same stripe.

The Doctor And The Lady

The lady might not trust men with beards. It might seem a long shot that she would ever fund a nutrition lab and clinic. Riordan was no specialist, though what he had seen of the effect of nutrition had impressed him, and people he admired — Pfeiffer and Pauling for example — were seriously committed to it. Yet he was a believer in destiny, was comfortable with change, was willing and able to act upon what he learned, and recognized opportunity when he met it. He was willing to credit dreams, and he believed in being quiet and listening to the way nature was taking things. He was, according to his own analysis, a perceiver, not a thinker. It was, he once said, very much "a part of my personality. It's a little old-countryish. I view it as the difference between making and allowing. Actually, everything in nature is pretty much an allowing thing. If you have a flower on an apple tree, you can't make an apple come out before it is ready to come out. If you don't try to make things happen you don't have the frustration that you didn't make it happen, which I think a lot of people feel."

Accordingly, he composed a hand-written note to the Garvey Foundation and its elderly scion. "You don't know what I am going to do," he said in essence, "and I do not know what I am going to do, but if you want to fund it, I'll devote three years of my life to making it work." Two weeks later he had the underwriting for the lab for three years.

"She was a gutsy person," Riordan always said. And so was he. It is difficult in hindsight to appreciate how far the so-called "Alternative" or "Holistic" medicine movement was from the mainstream in 1975. The trace mineral literature in which Riordan was interested had to be perused mostly in the veterinary textbooks. Ironically, nutrition was a big thing with valuable farm animals, but almost beside the point with people. Although the miracles of acute medical care, which Riordan deeply appreciated, had, by curing so many ailments, made chronic, metabolic disease ever more prominent among the problems of aging people, the idea that nutrition was a major influence on these was yet heresy. The American Cancer Society declared about that time that anyone who claimed nutrition might be among environmental factors contributing to the triggering and spread of cancers that might be contained potentially in genetic material was a quack. There was more respect for the role of diet and exercise in cardiovascular ailments, but still nothing like the attention that would be given it twenty years later. When Dr. Riordan tried at the hospital to get fresh fruit for his psychiatric patients, he was told that fruit came in #10 cans, and that they could not have that stuff rotting in the food preparation area. The only way Riordan could get it was by writing a prescription for it, and that he did.

The first patient from a substantial group of "hopeless" cases quickly referred by psychiatrists was seen by the new lab, located in a rented building near Hillside and Douglas on Wichita's near east side, on November 1, 1975, two months ahead of the planned schedule. It was the beginning of The Center for the Improvement of Human Functioning, which, by no accident, was, through several changes of its long name and twenty-five years of service, generally known to the public simply as the "Garvey Center."

It seemed a small enough step, but to take it merely for what it seemed at the time would have been a considerable mistake. For doubtless, more important than that Garvey provided Riordan with $300,000 in underwriting for the three year operation of a clinical nutritional/research laboratory was the fact that the funding began an association between two extraordinary people, both of whom were broad and unconventional thinkers who knew how to implement ideas and between them had the resources and expertise to do this in the field of alternative medicine. [9]

Though she was aware that "my [first] name was a symbol of surrender," Olive White Garvey had spent no time in her life being either withdrawn or ordinary. As a toddler she had pointed at a newspaper ad and said, "That spells 'shoes.'" She developed formidably. Her mother was 36 and her father 41 when she arrived, and as their girl rode her pony among the Kaw and Osage Indians on the family ranch in Indian Territory, they grounded her in the sensible, the humorous, and the wise. Her father was a considerable businessman in Topeka, and her neighbor there as a young woman was Charles Sheldon, who wrote the best-seller *In His Steps* and once edited the local paper for a week as he

---

9 See note 6.

thought it would be edited if Jesus were in charge. She earned a degree from Washburn University, taught school briefly, and then moved to western Kansas with her attorney husband. While Ray Garvey acquired businesses one after another and made them all work, Olive raised four children, painted, wrote, and increased the level of literary discourse among the local women, first in Colby and then in Wichita, where the family moved in 1928. There were crises and challenges all along, with which she calmly coped in her vigorous good health. "All worry," she once said, "is a very foolish, very neurotic waste of time."

Her early business experience consisted, she joked, of listening to one side of long-distance telephone conversations, but in 1959, at age 65, all that changed. She traveled to the East, where she charmed the bankers who had loaned her husband $50,000,000 to build grain elevators and wondered whether she could run them, and she kept a family of individualists together by ending meetings with her decision and the maxim from cartoonist Al Capp's Mammy Yokum that "I Has Spoke." Overshadowed perhaps for a time by her genius husband, she emerged in her own right as one of Wichita's influential "Olives," right there beside Olive Ann Beech, the chief executive of one of the nation's premier aircraft manufacturers. She was, in the words of the operating officer of her enterprise, "as strong as horseradish." There was no hesitation. "A woman must not indulge in feminine traits of temperament and emotion," she said. "And anyone in authority must be objective and judicious, particularly a woman."

She had changed careers late in life but had maintained her philosophy of practical local action in areas of human need. "Do that first which lies nearest thee," Thomas Carlyle had said. Olive often quoted that. And her thoroughgoing approach to things applied as much to her philanthropy and her hobbies as it did to her business. She clipped a cartoon of "Mr. Tweedy" in the 1960s, labeling it "self-portrait." It showed Tweedy putting up an easel in the park. Two men were standing by, one saying to the other: "If I ever decide to take up a hobby, I'm going to research it thoroughly rather than just muddle along blindly." The Riordan proposal for a nutritional laboratory let her combine her vision and her "creative work" with her pragmatic acumen.

There were many points at which her philosophy and Dr. Riordan's coincided. She liked Tolstoy's definition of art, which was "to make people *good* by *choice*...." That could apply as directly to Riordan' philosophy of decentralized wellness through individual responsibility. She had 300 years of Quakerism in two branches of her family, preparing her not only to be active as an independent woman, but to understand instinctively the doctor's philosophy of "allowing" rather than forcing change along the lines nature and nature's god dictated. She was a conservative and a radical at the same time also, just like him. He never abandoned his membership in the American Medical Association and never criticized standard medicine for doing the things it did best. He did not even like the term "alternative medicine," arguing that what he did was to complement standard medicine as it had developed over the ages, not replace it. Olive said similar things. Despite her free market, individualist philosophy, she did not consider herself a political conservative in the sense that it was popular to define that type in the 1960s, but rather a classical liberal. "The image of a conservative," she said, "is that he has a closed mind, but that isn't true. If we didn't have change, everything would be stagnant. But things have to be done in a logical order." Freedom, however, was to her freedom to change, "to venture, to initiate, to experiment and innovate.... You, only you, can make of yourself what you want." And she agreed strongly with Riordan about the holistic approach. Yes, Kirlian photography to record electric auras surrounding the body was great, and so was other medical technology. But it had to be applied to the "whole" person — "physical body, mental ability, and a pervading spirit." Thinking itself was hardly done in isolation. Thinking was, she wrote, "the ability to form abstract concepts and then test their authenticity against every actuality involved." Business had provided her with that kind of reality check, and certainly the new lab would also. "God does not live only in a church," wrote the woman who had sponsored the design and production of a major twentieth-century edition of the Bible, "He lives in me."[10]

Perhaps Garvey's most complete statement of her philosophy regard-

---

10 See note 1.

ing personal health came in a speech at Christian College in Oklahoma City in October, 1976, entitled "The Wholistic Me." Olive was there to receive one of her four honorary doctorates, but also to give young people some advice from a woman born in 1893. She had a friend, she said, who was a practicing psychiatrist (that would be Dr. Riordan) who said that the human race had not yet learned to think. Much had been accomplished in the area of manual dexterity. The younger generation had inherited more knowledge than any other generation in history, but too many of them lacked the maturity and skill to correlate and apply it. World history was a sad story, she thought, of the return of problems that had come and gone before, including, prominently, senseless wars. "It seems that even to the present time our world is without understanding of the causes of our troubles and without a comprehensive plan to cure them." Blaming "them" was no solution. "Let me tell you something. 'We' and 'they' are the same. We all emerge as 'me' and 'me' is all for which I am responsible. 'They,' that faceless mass known as society, is not an entity. It is an accumulation of you and me and everybody else."

Health was essential.

> I coin the term 'Wholistic: I am composed of body, mind and spirit working together. How does such a Me work? Although my body is lent to me as my habitation while in this world, it is dependent upon my mental processes to preserve it. There are certain instincts which have preserved life from time immemorial. But modern situations require more than instinct. They require thought, intelligence. Is it intelligent to eat foods which do not properly nourish? Is indolence intelligent? Is it intelligent to use drugs which hamper my body's development, or alcohol which clouds my mind, or tobacco which threatens dread disease? Is it conceivable that people think, who in the face of all the knowledge available are actually increasing the use of these poisons?

The mind and spirit suffered from a malfunctioning body. "Learning, energy, ambition, general well-being are dependent on the body's health." Personality and stability were affected by diet, and balance allowed people to make a living and to establish satisfactory social relationships. Young people did not get good foods in the normal course of events, and that was a tragedy. "The body is basic to life; the mind determines the pursuits and judgments of one's lifetime." Better diet could prevent "the break-up of homes" which has "become an epidemic bordering on a pestilence." So could thinking ahead, which required whole health. Olive's sociology teacher advised on marriage to "Judge before loving, then confide until death." She herself saw too many people in their 30s "still wallowing in a philosophical morass" and "still engaged in the adolescent pursuit of 'finding themselves.'" Maturity and wholeness, health and rationality were the key — so simple and yet requiring a great change in the way people treated their bodies and consequently their souls. It was not just a matter of junk food vs. vitamins; it was the basis of a social revolution.[11]

Hugh Riordan gave a talk just two months later entitled "A Humanistic Approach to Medical Practice" which paralleled Garvey's philosophy in many ways. The doctor and the patient, he said, had to have a personal as well as a formal relationship, and the patient needed to understand and be understood as a whole person. A patient was not a bundle of symptoms or an example of disease, not a symbol of youth or old age, "but a concrete person before my eyes." And that person was unique and rare. "Each of us," he observed, "assuming an ordinary conception, out swam 300-400 million sperm, overcoming incredible odds, with which we are never faced again, except at our time of demise." Dr. Riordan's mother had tried to breast feed him according to the clock, every four hours, and "only by pointers affixed to a mechanical device that had never needed human milk for nourishment." What a non-humanistic, non-holistic approach.

Never deny a patient his symptoms, Riordan's mentor and early

---

11 Olive Garvey, "The Wholistic Me," printed pamphlet, Oct. 18, 1976, in History Scrapbook #1, CIHF Archives.

Wichita medical partner Fowler Poling had told him. Never blame the patient. "How preposterous and demeaning it is to tell a 65-year-old gentleman that he has bad veins — when those veins have been carrying his blood for 65 years." The doctor's humanness was not enhanced when others were demeaned through his activities. Why emphasize sickness more than wellness? Why separate the injured part from the person, as though doing surgery through a hole in a sheet? It was important to see "patients not just as they are but such as they are." An injured child felt his entire being was injured. It was important to tell him what was hurt and what was not. Self-image was a part of healing, as much as knowledge, and even the knowledge was something that must be shared by the healed as well as the healer. Even such a simple act as the placement of a needle or catheter in a patient sent a message to the entire self and affected the healing process in ways quite independent of the specific treatment. It was a contact between two complete humans, it was complex, and it must be understood and respected fully. He must, he said, see the subject "as a feeling, thinking human being and secondly as an organism with pathological problems."[12] Allowing patients to get to know him was a risk: they might not like him. But Riordan, who called himself an SOB (defined as "sunny old bird"), thought it was an absolute essential.

He was glad to be called a humanist in the most traditional sense. "I really like people," Riordan said to a reporter early in the evolution of The Center, "probably because I like myself so well — so I always find something good in everyone. Negativism is very bad, and easily transferable to patients. This may blow your mind, but I'm a religious man. I thank God every day — several times a day — for allowing me 'to be.' But I find prayer requests inappropriate. God must be saying, 'I gave you life, now you're asking for more. What else do you want?'"[13]

Certainly Hugh Riordan was a match for Olive Garvey, both in background and vision, and the two without question interested and

---

12 Hugh Riordan, "A Humanistic Approach to Medical Practice" printed in *Dialogue* (Dec, 1976): 6-8 in History Scrapbook #1, CIHF Archives.
13 "The Humanistic Shrink," *The Wichitan* (Dec, 1978), in ibid.

admired each other very much. At first their relationship was mostly philosophical, developing in a series of hand-written notes and letters. But later Riordan became her personal physician. She wouldn't follow the rules of the clinic by submitting a full medical history, but Riordan was able to make educated guesses, based on laboratory findings about her ailments which turned out to be accurate and increased her confidence in him. She recommended him to friends and communicated with him eventually about her most personal hopes and fears, from spiritualism to backache. He much appreciated her also, especially that "she never interfered with anything," never intervened in any fundamental way in the day-to-day affairs of The Center that she was financing, though she was hardly shy about expressing her opinions to Hugh personally. Riordan attributed her attitude both to the fact that even during the first years of the lab it had nearly paid its way, requiring less than the full amount of her underwriting, and that he reported regularly to her on the progress, something she told him several times no other beneficiaries of Garvey Foundation largesse had ever done until they needed more money.[14] Riordan was with her when she died at age 99 in 1993, and she said matter-of-factly shortly before that final event that she thought Dr. Riordan could keep her alive forever, but she did not want him to.[15]

Like her, he came to that day in 1975 by a long path and hardly entered that new enterprise naive or inexperienced. His office was no more standard than Olive Garvey's. In 1981, it was described as a "cross between a magician's lair and a child's playroom." It was lit by a "soft, windowless incandescence," and included a trampoline behind his desk, a paper kite hanging from the wall, and a tree seeming to grow out of the wall.[16] Updating that description to 1998, one would have to change "windowless" to "lit by skylight from above," and maybe substitute "kettle drum" for "kite," but as The Center grew and Riordan's job became more like that of a major company CEO, the appearance

---

14 Interview, Hugh Riordan with Craig Miner, May 27, 1998.
15 Letter, Riordan to Olive Garvey, January 26, 1992, Office Files, CIHF Archives.
16 *Salina Journal,* Nov 4, 1981 in History Scrapbook #1, CIHF Archives.

of his office had less and less in common with the standard, and, he would say, intimidating and inhuman, environs of others of his ilk.

Riordan's presence was always formidable before he ever opened his mouth. He was tall, about 6'3" with a heavy frame and large feet. Many were reminded of a bear. He once described himself as "big, bald, bearded and blue." He thought he might be a descendent of Genghis Khan on his mother's side. He certainly was a descendent of one of Napoleon's generals (from whom he took his middle name) and of Russians and Irish.[17]

And he could, as he would put it, "shift gears." Once he attracted kids all over the neighborhood to his yard by bringing in a six-foot pile of dirt and then letting their imaginations go to work.[18] When he did not like the food at the airport restaurant in Dodge City, where he was flying for consulting, he leased the place and made money selling better food to others. He had not been in full psychiatric practice since 1967, having moved some of his time into communications consulting. That was due to the need to redefine his mission at midlife and to move away from administrative responsibilities and back into direct patient care. He took John Gardner's advice seriously that it was good for people in middle life to take some time off and rethink themselves. In 1967 he decided to organize his life so as never again to do professionally what he did not enjoy doing. "I've since then structured my life to enjoy what I'm doing," he said in 1983. "I'm sure that's a mystery to many people who set their pattern and stick with it. But I'm also convinced that many would like to do something different — like I did then."[19]

His family background read like a novel of high adventure. Louis Charles Antoine Desaix de Veygoux was born in France in 1768, joined Napoleon's army, and was a general by 1800. He became governor of France's North African and Egyptian colonies. After wresting victory from defeat for Napoleon in the Italian campaign of 1800, he was killed

---

17 The Humanistic Shrink," *The Wichitan* (Dec, 1976), in ibid.
18 *Wichita Beacon,* April 23, 1980.
19 "The Humanistic Shrink," *The Wichitan* (Dec, 1976), History Scrapbook #1, CIHF Archives.

at age 32. The general's great granddaughter, Tatiana Alexandropol, a girl with a mix of French, Russian, German and Mongolian blood, by labyrinthine twists of fate, ended up in St. Petersburg. Caught in the Russian revolution, she, at age 19 and with a good education behind her, was chosen by her family to escape to the East. She traveled across Siberia in a cattle car, arriving first in Vladivastok and then in Japan so penniless that for a considerable while she nearly starved, surviving on bananas.[20]

But there was a way in which she was the lucky one. She heard years later that all the rest of her family had been killed.[21] She supported herself by giving French lessons in Tokyo, and one of her students was an economics professor at the University of Tokyo named Hugh Riordan. The two fell in love, and their lives seemed charmed. In 1923 there was a serious earthquake in Japan. Tatiana that day was scheduled to go from Tokyo to Yokohama by train. She missed it. Everyone on the train was killed. The hotel where Professor Riordan lived collapsed, but he had taken refuge under a stone arch and survived. For some hours each presumed the other was dead. Reunited, they went through Ceylon, married in Nice, France, and became the parents of Lee and Hugh Desaix Riordan, the latter of whom in the 1970s was embarking on an adventure of his own in Kansas.[22]

Since his father was the youngest of 16 children, the younger Hugh Riordan was to be "unencumbered by grandparents." But he was the beneficiary of a rich tradition. The toilet in his Milwaukee apartment was called a "benjo" — the Japanese word— and there was much of oriental wisdom in his childhood play that dated from the time his parents met in Japan. This was mixed with his father's European background, and the influence of the French people who would visit the home due to the elder Mr. Riordan's role as French consul in Milwaukee. There were failures, of course, in transferring culture. Riordan's father was, for example, eager that he should play the violin, even hoped he would be

---

20 Typed biography of Hugh Riordan, n.d. (1984), History Scrapbook #1(a), ibid.
21 Interview, Dr. Hugh Riordan with Craig Miner, May, 20, 1998.
22 Typed biography of Hugh Riordan, n.d. (1984), History Scrapbook #1(a), ibid.

a great violinist, "but after two years of my screeching, he realized the error of his ways."

The rest of his upbringing was perhaps not so unusual except that the extraordinary little boy made it so. Hugh did not start school until age seven. He credited this with his having developed a firm sense of self before ever venturing beyond his solid family into the sometimes critical world. "I knew I was OK before I got to school, though I don't know what OK meant. I didn't have a lot of fears and stuff like that." He remembered that "everything was smooth growing up. Maybe because we lived on the third floor, I don't know, and felt protected." More likely it was the confidence and optimism of his parents, having overcome so much. "It seemed to me," the son recalled, "that the concept was 'We'll find a way' to do something." There were lots of good family stories, and they were all true.

He went to pubic school, skipping a grade or two. He was second string center on the football team in high school, worked on the annual and spoke at the graduation. The family home was three blocks from Lake Michigan, and the streets were a kind of playground for creative boys. Hugh and a his friend Duane Quintal often visited the city dump, where they scavenged wonderful things on "gold mine Saturdays" to use in their electronics projects. With another friend, Roger Reinke, Hugh would listen to the police radio and arrive at accident scenes to take photographs, which they would sell to the press. Half of the pantry in the Riordan apartment was Hugh's "command center." There was a crystal radio set there and a little microscope, but the early emphasis was on electricity, not biology.

His career in business began by mowing lawns at age thirteen, shortly combining with another boy in a considerable mowing and trimming business. Later jobs were unusually varied. In high school he worked for the husband of one of his lawn customers at Northwest Furniture as a switchboard operator while participating in wrestling, shot put, and football in school. In High School he won the Harvard Book Award and had a scholarship to attend there. He could also have gone to Marquette University free, since his father was a professor there. But he did neither ("dumb, dumb, dumb," he said in hindsight half seriously). He wanted to work and to live at home, and he learned much by attending the University of Wisconsin at Milwaukee for two years (that was all that was offered then in the city) and attending classes in a four-story building downtown. He transferred to the main campus at Madison to receive his degree there. He took a challenging load of courses, was elected prom king, and balanced his life with a series of jobs.

The jobs were interesting. He worked for a year after high school at Taylor Electric, where he was trained by IBM in Chicago. He went about with Taylor's top salesman, learning all about what motivated people to buy appliances. As a freshman at the University of Wisconsin at Milwaukee he worked for the controller of the Fox Theater. He had to go to a movie every night, partly because he, with his size, acted as a sort of security system in case there was trouble. He saw *Gentlemen Prefer Blondes* 22 times. It was there he learned "instant hypnotic techniques" that resulted from saying and doing incongruous things and bewildering people. Once a group of three or four ganged up on Hugh in a restroom. He simply said "I eat guys like you for breakfast every day," and that was apparently sufficiently bewildering that they backed off. So effective was he that he later became a bouncer at George Divine's Million Dollar Ballroom, dealing most effectively with sailors who got out of control. Later when he was accosted by a man with a gun outside a locked mental patient area at St. Francis Hospital in Wichita, Riordan said, "Give me the gun or I'll kill you." Another instant hypnosis.

Another particularly interesting job during college, probably also at first related to his size, was at the Bjorksten Research Labs. Dr. Bjorksten had invented many things, including much of the technology for a liquid pencil that evolved into the ball-point pen, and was in demand for applied technological research. The work there involved government contracts and was top secret. Riordan had to carry a gun. In what he calls "probably my most disturbed period," Riordan ignored the billboards advising people not to pick up hitchhikers by picking up every one he saw, the "sleazier the better." He had a Beretta concealed on his left ankle and secretly hoped some hitchhiker would try something, but, although it was rumored that one in four of these people were criminals, none ever made the slightest threat. Riordan's tenure there was largely without incident, except that one night he failed to report in to the sheriff, as he was to do hourly. He had fallen asleep on Dr. Bjorksten's huge desk and was awakened about 5:30 a.m. by his boss and three sheriff's officers. He thought that job was over, but all Bjorksten said was that it would be nice if he could remain awake while at work.

While in Madison, Riordan managed the apartment building where he lived for the widowed owner, whose husband had invented the super heterodyne (AM) radio. This otherwise charming woman had the annoying habit of knocking only after her key was already in the door and then bursting suddenly into the room. Riordan and his roommate decided they would "alter Mrs. Wengel's behavior." Therefore, one day at about the time she generally popped in on them, they lounged about the living room totally naked. Her behavior pattern was broken that day.

Medical School was at the University of Wisconsin also, and Hugh married Jan Brick, a nurse, in his junior year. He was always a little uncertain why he changed his interest from engineering to medicine, but his interest in psychiatry was certainly partly an accident. During medical school, he worked at the Wisconsin Diagnostic Center, which, when he applied, he thought was a cancer research lab, but was actually a psychiatric center. He learned later that his 40 hour a week job at The Center violated some of the school's rules concerning outside work for students, and the exact manner that they should proceed with their education. Riordan was once quoted on the front page of the local newspaper about his work and called before a dean who had been head of medical operations in the European Theater in World War II and was not sympathetic to individual variations on the system.[23] Hugh did not bother to tell him about his interest in African drum music or his deal with the keeper of the school cadavers to trade a fifth of bourbon for a gallon of ethyl in order for a classmate to manufacture gin by

---

23 Interview, Hugh Riordan with Craig Miner, May 20, 1998.

distillation.[24] The Dean told him as a parting comment, "I'll flunk you if I can."[25]

Out of these early experiences in life came several strong personal characteristics. For one thing, he was basically an optimist. In medical school he and classmates were shown a picture of a monkey leaping for a tree with a lion about to close his mouth on one of his feet. Riordan was the only one commenting on the picture who thought the monkey would get away. "I'm a very big believer in expectations," he says, "If you have expectations, they have a lot to do with how things turn out." That is much in contrast to the majority of the population who, if asked how people who do not know them might identify them, usually come up with some aberration or negative characteristic instead of a candid description of themselves. "I did not have that growing up," Riordan notes. There were not "universal pats on the back," but there was never the notion from his parents that he was stupid or that he could not do something. "I think it's a lot more fun being a realistic optimist." Certainly that trait helped him with The Center. When asked how essential he was to The Center, he said not essential at all in the 1990s, but in the beginning he was probably essential because he was the only one around, except Mrs. Garvey, who really believed The Center would work.

A second helpful characteristic, derived doubtless from upbringing and early experience, was an ability to focus on one thing at a time and not to fret needlessly over things that could not be changed, or could not be changed right away. Riordan always had many interests. When he moved the psychiatric practice after the death of Fowler Poling in 1967, he, with scarcely a hitch, expanded his audio-visual company and began consulting by airplane in western Kansas and with various clinics. Change seemed normal to him, as it does with so many entrepreneurs, and he was more eager for and stimulated by new things than he was nostalgic for past patterns. "It is nothing for me to walk out of one room and into another," he said, "and totally leave what was in

---

24 Ibid, June 10, 1998.
25 Ibid, October 22, 1998.

that room." There were no lingering thoughts in going from one thing to another; it was just "going through a doorway." Of course he was filled with ideas, but ideas are not enough without the personal ability to walk through the door into a future that might include implementation of a dream but is also fraught with risk. Riordan thought of it as "shifting gears," and liked people who could do it. "I don't know if it's so much entrepreneurship," he said, "as just being interested in things. I guess if you're interested in things that are not currently there, that automatically makes you an entrepreneur." New ideas are ideas for which there are no peers, and those with new ideas can be frustrated people in seeking any support from an establishment based on old ideas. But it was Riordan's nature not only to have new ideas but to feel secure in the change, and even amid the criticism that came from pursuing them. That meeting with Garvey in 1975 was a door into a room he had glimpsed but never before entered. Yet he had no hesitation in turning the key.

His "allowing" mode included always time in the day for a sort of meditation, where strength was gathered. Meditation was not "chanting mantras" for him, but quiet time to listen to nature speak. At The Center for the Improvement of Human Functioning there was an hour long lunch break rather than a half hour, and that was on purpose so that employees could take a walk, "lie down and read," or otherwise break up their day by thinking creatively about non-programmed things. "To me," according to Riordan, "one of the most delightful things is to watch the sunset, to watch it get dark without electronic interference.... I may work 75 hours a week, but part of that is put aside for what I call input, which means that I am alone and information or whatever it is I want to have come my way or filter through has time." They are lessons from elsewhere, from what both he and Olive Garvey would call the spiritual realm.[26]

But Riordan was no passive guru. "I think the serenity prayer is pretty good," he said, "but there are things you can change."[27] He

---

26 Ibid, May 20, 1998.
27 Interview, Hugh Riordan with Craig Miner, June 6, 1998,

was a doer, and not everything he did sat well with those whose livings were threatened. Not everyone understood or admired Riordan, making it all the more remarkable that Garvey would back him. But Ray Garvey, respected as he was, was hardly mainstream either, and the family was no stranger to criticism from self-assured if unimaginative second-guessers ensconced in the status quo. Perhaps that created empathy.

Riordan had controversial methods as a psychiatrist. He could be blunt, even shocking. Once this exchange was reported: "Dr. Riordan: 'So what are you going to do with your life?' Female Patient: 'I don't know [looking glum].' Dr. Riordan: 'Why don't you be a prostitute?' Female Patient: [gasp] 'How could you say something like that?' Dr. Riordan: 'Well, that way you could *really* hurt your parents. Isn't that what you're trying to do?'" On another occasion, he met a lonely woman at a party who went home feeling depressed. He called her and told her to get herself back there and suggested she have a good time. She did.

His supporters called him a "tender, caring" man; his critics called him "an eccentric flake" on the lunatic fringe. He himself often joked later that when he started The Center he was considered "100% quack" and over the years advanced to maybe "25% quack." Other doctors who were interviewed about him at the time The Center opened often said they could not decide for sure whether Riordan was "twenty years ahead of his time or completely out in left field." One said: "He's a one-man show, with methods that are not scientific enough for me." Another: "He's a fadist with the reputation of not completing projects, not carrying through." Another: "A very intelligent man who is always going off on a tangent from the rest of the world. But who knows, he may be right. Fifty years from now, what he's doing may be the whole 'schmear.' He's a knowledgeable practitioner." Another: "A workaholic, and frustrating to work with at times, but very exciting. He's an idea man who refuses to be locked into one pattern of thinking." Another: "Hugh is a long-time professional friend, and I've watched him evolve. He may be too 'rich for my blood,' but I don't think he can be written off. After all, when Newton's apple dropped, nobody was thinking of gravity."[28] Still another: "I like Hugh personally, he's always been kind of a flamboyant guy. But some of us are kind of uncomfortable with some of what he's doing — and I guess some of us wish we'd gotten to Mrs. Garvey first."[29] All concurred that he had, as well as many detractors, a "fantastic minority of vigorous supporters." They would quote with their mentor the maxim that "While they were saying it couldn't be done, it was done."[30]

It was obvious from the start that the thinking of both Riordan and Garvey extended well beyond the modest experimental lab they had established to consult with mental health patients. In January 1976, for example, Riordan reported to the Garvey Foundation on a dream that he had while attending a seminar in Phoenix. "In this dream," he wrote, "a concept for a Wichita-based international health center closely allied with nutrition as the most important facet unfolded with great clarity." His mission, glimpsed in the dream, was providing leadership in the field of human nutrition "because public opinion follows leaders more than it follows evidence. I was to be the one providing leadership because I had swum upstream against the current for many years and, therefore, had demonstrated my stamina in such circumstances."

He intended now to "desensitize opponents that appear rather than confront them, since he could grasp the concept that "the mind reacts to a new idea much as the body reacts to a foreign protein."

During his dream, Riordan got the message that he should phase out fee for service office activity and receive only a salary from The Center. He was to form a new department to be associated with a medical institution of higher learning (Wichita had just gotten a medical school branch) called the "Department of Biomedical Brainstorm." This would provide the nucleus for a TV series to be called *Biomedical Brainstorm* and for a journal and seminars on how to care for oneself.

---

28 "The Humanist Shrink," *The Wichitan* (Dec., 1978) in History Scrapbook #1, CIHF Archives.
29 Angelia Herrin, "Trying to Go Beyond," *Evening Eagle Beacon* (Wichita), Sept. 5, 1982, ibid.
30 "The Humanist Shrink," *The Wichitan* (Dec., 1978) in History Scrapbook #1, ibid.

The Center would evolve from the traditional concept of medicine with its concern for function, structure, and chemistry to the broader concept of function, structure, biochemistry, energy field, and mind. A disturbance in any of these fields caused "perturbations throughout," and what was needed was "a system of therapy and prevention which deals with all segments sequentially or simultaneously. The essential construct here is that if there is pathology at one level there is pathology at all levels including the mind. Thus we would operate on the premise that if the body or the mind is unable to receive the whole spectrum of energy there cannot be total health."

Structurally he imagined that The Center for the Improvement of Human Functioning would have a lab called the Brain Bio Center, one for Biochemical Research, one for Kirlian Phenomenon, one for Cytotoxic Evaluation, and others focusing on cybernetics, auricular medicine, nutritional therapy and amino acid evaluation." There would be an "Internal State Section" and an "External State Section," the latter to "develop as our understanding increased our level of awareness of extra corporal energies." He imagined moving out of the series of small buildings in which The Center started to a location on an organic farm, which could supply nutritional ingredients for research and short term treatment, as well as including a guest house for visiting lecturers. Riordan personally would put all his energies into it. "Just as the sun's rays can be focused by a magnifying glass to ignite a combustible into flame, so can a concept properly and intensively focused light a flame for the betterment of mankind." To do so, he wrote, "I must professionally put my head on the block and take the risk."

He had told Mrs. Garvey it might take 7-9 years to convince the scoffers. Personally he only hoped it would not take 79 years. But he would document every step. There would be attacks, but no turning back, since, as another of Riordan's collection of maxims had it, "Once you know something you cannot not know it." Garvey, with her faith in "next year country" born of watching western Kansas weather and the wheat, had set things in motion. "The mind is everything. You have studied the body, you have learned that the flow of energy of one person can profoundly effect another person — now discover that the mind is everything and you will discover how to prevent unnecessary disease. You have the capacity to see what others have not seen because you have felt the energy."[31]

That level of speculation at that time, had it been made public, would have caused those establishment figures who could not learn what they thought they already knew to rub their hands with glee at Riordan's foolish temerity. It doubtless would have given some of his supporters pause enough to say something like, "I agree with you on most things, but...." However, with Mrs. Garvey, Dr. Riordan found a person with whom to explore whatever seemed feasible, not in the ordinary world, but in the special world her vision and support could create, if not indefinitely sustain. Should there have been any need to document that individual human beings are biochemically and holistically unique, the study could have begun and ended with this field of two. This man in his mid-forties and this woman in her mid-eighties started off into the unknown that day in the mid-seventies on the Great Plains with as steady a step as though they were idealistic youths who did not know what was likely to strike them. That they did know, and acted anyway, according to their hopes and not their fears, made all the difference.

---

[31] Hugh Riordan to Cliff Allison, Jan. 4, 1976, Correspondence Files, CIHF Archives.

Chapter Two
Throwing A Rope

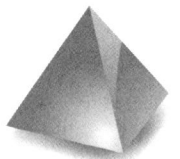

Dr. Riordan joked often about the lack of a grand plan in the development of The Center for the Improvement of Human Functioning. "The whole place," he would say, "has kind of evolved as if it were meant to be."

Whatever the long-range thinking, the original Garvey commitment was for three years of underwriting of a nutritional and clinical laboratory, and maximum funding of $300,000. Since it was funded out of an annuity which she received for her lifetime, Olive sometimes joked that Hugh better keep her living. Mrs. Garvey was not only pleased that Riordan kept her informed about his progress, but also her business side was gratified that there was market demand for the clinical services to the extent that the original test project made a substantial part of its own way, and drew far less than the authorized funding from the Garvey Foundation. But from Riordan's perspective there was considerable uncertainty. Since the underwriting depended on the income and the income varied, checks from the foundation did not come in regularly. The staff expenses were always paid, but Riordan's salary, down considerably anyway from what he had once earned in full-time, busy psychiatric practice, was where the flexibility was, and "I never knew whether I would get paid or not."

Riordan's office was at 434 N. Oliver, where he had located in the early 1960s in private practice. The Center shortly expanded into some adjoining duplexes. The lab, named the Bio Center Laboratory, was in the building at 3715 E. Douglas, formerly occupied by an osteopathic practice. Riordan had a busy hospital practice with the psychiatric patients who came to him, but the lab began supplementing the usual hospital procedures with tests that sought nutritional solutions. During the first year, 86% of the patients at first were physician referrals. Initially the approach was based on Dr. Pfeiffer's work, which included knowledge that some mentally ill people excreted pyrroles in the urine, which led to a zinc and vitamin B6 deficiency that was related to their illness. Other factors, such as polyamines and the neurotransmitter, histamine, were subjects of interest in relation to psychiatric problems.[1]

The national news indicated there was some reason to believe such a direction was becoming better accepted in certain circles. In the fall of 1976 Dr. Arnold Schaefer of Omaha, director of the Swanson Center for Nutrition, said that if doctors were better trained in nutrition they would be the "first line against food quackery." He advised that nutrition be made a major part of the curriculum in medical schools. His center sponsored a two-day symposium on nutrition in pediatrics attended by representatives of ten medical schools.

Dr. Myron Winick, professor of nutrition and pediatrics at Columbia University commented that this addressed a considerable lack in traditional medical education. Good nutrition would help prevent illness but it was difficult to establish a "hard cause and effect relationship between nutrition and particular medical results." When a doctor used penicillin, the result was obvious and immediate. "With nutrition, we have a good idea what will happen but except for very clear situations, the doctor isn't on as firm scientific grounds as he is with many other things."[2]

Perhaps as influential as anything in the national news was the

---

[1] Interview, Dr. Hugh Riordan with Craig Miner, May 27, 1998, October 22, 1998.
[2] *Omaha World Herald* in *Rope*, Sept. 17, 1976.

publicity on an article in the December 1976 issue of the prestigious *New England Journal of Medicine* by Norman Cousins. It was called "Anatomy of an Illness (as Perceived by the Patient)." The main point that was picked up by the media was Cousins' claim that he had in 1964 literally laughed his way out of a serious illness (ankylosing spondylitis) by watching comedy on his hospital TV and reading humorous books. That by itself was useful to places like The Center for the Improvement of Human Functioning (CIHF) in suggesting that illness was holistic and that attitude might be part of the healing process. But Cousins in the original piece had some other very interesting things to say about medicine and about his treatment that were not widely reported. One of them was to criticize the sad state of hospital nutrition, calling the profusion of processed foods with preservatives and harmful dyes which he was served there "inexcusable." A second point often overlooked in the popular coverage was that Cousins convinced his doctor to stop all drugs and to give him instead high doses of intravenous vitamin C, far beyond any dose the hospital had ever given. In fact he had to leave the hospital to get it. No one there seemed to think it would have any effect, but since Cousins' disease had offered only a 1 in 500 chance of recovery, why not? Cousins had done some reading, including a book by Walter Cannon called *The Wisdom of the Body*, and Hans Seyle's *The Stress of Life*, and he thought perhaps his illness was caused by heavy metals from the polluted environment of the Soviet Union, where he had recently spent some time. The resulting adrenal exhaustion could, he thought, be helped by positive emotions (thus the laughter) and also by the vitamin C. And last, he emphasized he felt he had to get out of the hospital to have any chance of getting well.

Cousins recovered. He was only one person. Science was not impressed, but the public was. Here was an intelligent man who had taken control of his own health regimen, and with a couple of techniques, one very old, one newer, had cured himself. Just maybe there was some wisdom outside of hospitals. He wrote that: "Living in the second half of the twentieth century, I realized, confers no automatic protection against unwise or even dangerous drugs and methods. Each age has to undergo its own special nostrums. Fortunately, the human body is a remarkably durable instrument and has been able to withstand all sorts of prescribed assaults over the centuries."[3]

Reaching a broader audience also, thanks partly to the new Wichita Center, was the work of Dr. Roger Williams. His book *The Wonderful World Within You* (1977) was, in 1987, the first publication of The Center's Bio-Communications Press. The Press was a pioneer effort in desk-top publishing, and the book was perfect for it — so perfect that The Center reprinted it again in 1998, updated and in fancier dress.

"How one fares in old age," Williams wrote in that book, "may depend on how well one has prepared in youth and middle age. One of the tragedies of middle and old age is failure to recognize that illnesses do not arise out of nothing. People who are visited with sickness late in life often have no idea they may have been paving the way for years."[4] There was a unity in life. The child indeed was father to the man. And there was an interdependence of factors that must be recognized.

The body was complex. It had 60 trillion cells, each composed of 1 quadrillion molecules — 10,000 times as many as the Milky Way had stars. That made everyone a "person of parts." Yet there were limits too. The reproduction of nerve cells stopped at birth, and when one was a year old, one had as many brain cells as he or she would ever have. Nerve cells took ten times the nourishment of other cells, and all cells were complex in organization, much more so than a watch or a TV set. They had their own power plants and waste disposal systems and could build other cells. No wonder that poor nourishment could impair a personality as well as a physique.

Each species of organism required a distinctive set of maintenance chemicals. The modern tragedy was that humankind had moved from eating plant and animal tissues to other foods. Macaroni, Williams pointed out, is not a vegetable.

---

[3] Norman Cousins, "Anatomy of an Illness (as Perceived by the Patient)," *New England Journal of Medicine*, Dec. 23, 1976, vol. 295, no 26.
[4] Roger J. Williams, *The Wonderful World Within You* (Wichita: Bio-Communications Press, 1987), ix.

Every individual was different. Stomachs varied in size and shape, in their quantity of digestive juices, and in the placement of their valves.[5] "People exhibit marked differences in the ways they walk, run, talk, breathe, write, throw a ball, play tennis or play golf."[6] The way their muscles are attached to their bones differed, whether they could open or close certain fingers independently varied. Robert Schumann was miserable for years because a normal characteristic of his hands prevented him from becoming a piano virtuoso. Thyroid glands varied six times in size among different individuals, as did sex glands and the number of islets in the pancreas producing insulin. Pain receptors varied widely in sensitivity, so much so that the test for witches once was whether their hands were insensitive to pain. Some professional boxers are relatively insensitive to pain. "Each individual has to adapt to his or her own system."[7]

To Williams that was wonderful. "Nature has made it impossible for you to have a pancake personality, without distinctive form, color, or markings. Nature has made you something like a multi-colored distinctive marble, something that cannot be averaged." We are a mystery even to those closest to us, and often to ourselves.[8]

Williams was exactly Olive Garvey's age. Both were born in 1893 (she in July, he in August). Williams lived to be 94 and Garvey 99.[9] Both made significant contributions in the field of nutrition when in their 80s. Williams noticed that the queen bee lived seven years when fed royal jelly, while female workers on a different diet lived only a few weeks. He cured his own leg cramps and some vision problems when in his 80s by applying the results of 2,000 hours he spent in the library looking up nutritional effects. Nutrition was not simple. Eggs contained cholesterol, but also were high in lechitin which prevented its deposit in the veins. Milk was high in some nutrients, but low in iron,

---

5 Ibid, pp. 11-12, 20-21, 52, 66.
6 Ibid, p. 68.
7 Ibid, pp. 69-74.
8 Ibid, p. 96.
9 Interview, Dr. Don Davis with Craig Miner, June 17, 1998.

copper and chromium. What he proposed was a science to be sure, but a science based on nature.[10]

To The Center, it was time to build on such thoughts. A year into the initial three, it started a circular letter to the Garvey Foundation and other supporters called "Throwing a Rope." The first such letter was produced the first week of October 1976 and provided "inside detail" on daily operations. The name appeared in 1979. The title was appropriate in two ways. First, just as The Center held the philosophy that patients should be "co-learners," fully informed about what was being done to and with them and why, so should financial supporters know exactly what they were supporting. Second, The Center in its first years was certainly trying to "throw a rope" to the mainstream medical profession and its institutions. Not only was cooperation philosophically appropriate, but there seemed no financial possibility to establish a self-standing alternative medicine center without considerable income from grants initiated by others, from lab work done for others, from credit courses in cooperation with universities, from patients referred by others, and from insurance payments typical of the standard medical system. It was only after considerable frustration in attempting to establish such connections, and after numerous "throws," that a plan and backing emerged for a more ambitious and more independent operation for an institution that was either too far ahead or too far to one side of the mainstream to slide comfortably into an established niche.

The staff was always a critical element, and the small group that found itself at the various Center locations was well-suited to the work. The earliest major staff member of that first three year experience was Dr. Charles Hinshaw, who was medical director of the laboratory and commuted from Hutchinson. Dr. Hinshaw and Dr. Riordan met in a revealing experience together. Riordan had been acting as a political consultant and was attending a Republican dinner in Topeka. During the event there was a medical emergency, for which a doctor was called. There were numerous specialists there, many internists and surgeons, but the only ones who responded were Riordan and Hinshaw, a psychi-

---

10 Williams, *Wonderful World*, pp. 145-49, 205.

atrist and a pathologist. Riordan thought that it illustrated the lack of confidence specialists had in their generalized understanding of health, as well as their lack of cardiopulmonary resuscitation techniques.

Later at a medical meeting Riordan, recalling the Topeka episode, suggested that all physicians in the Sedgwick County Medical Society take CPR training. The reaction to his "throwing a rope" was a "tar and feather episode." The physicians were not going to have any "ambulance guy" teaching them. Riordan responded that no one knew everything and it was best to learn from someone knowledgeable. His conclusion, however, was that "without their accoutrements and whatever they hang out they (physicians) were not comfortable doing something."[11] That Dr. Hinshaw was comfortable with it led to an association and to Hinshaw's working part time, at some financial sacrifice, running The Center's lab. CPR retraining subsequently became a regular feature of the training of people employed by The Center.

Another early staff member in the lab was Shu-Jen Chang Yeh, PhD, who ran the lab day to day. Her doctorate was in nutritional biochemistry from the University of Illinois, her husband had taken a job at Cessna in Wichita, and she came to The Center in August 1975, right at the outset. Yeh set up the lab, determined its methods and equipped and trained the first staff before the arrival of Hinshaw allowed her to turn her attention to research more than clinical tests.[12] In the spring of 1977, the lab got the highest possible rating from the Communicable Disease Center on three blind samples sent to them for evaluation.[13] In 1978 Yeh's husband was reassigned to Wright-Patterson Air Force Base in Dayton, Ohio, and she resigned her position at The Center. She would be missed, the *Rope* said, because of her "fine scientific mind," because of her "wonderful congeniality," and because "nutritional biochemists are not a very common find in this part of the country."[14] Tragically, Dr. Yeh died of cardiac arrest during elective

---

11 Interview, Dr. Hugh Riordan with Craig Miner, May 20, 1998.
12 Staff Profiles, CIHF Archives.
13 *Rope*, March 11, 1977.
14 Ibid, Jan. 9, 1978.

surgery in Dayton in 1980. Dr. Riordan attended the funeral on behalf of The Center.[15]

Sharon Authenreith (later Neathery) came late in 1975, as the first laboratory tech to be hired. She performed the cytotoxic tests for food sensitivities, as she had learned in St. Louis with Dr. George Ulett. This introduced a novel procedure in the Wichita area. In 2000, Sharon, after Dr. Riordan, had the record for seniority as a Center employee. She still specialized in the cytotoxic test.[16]

Brenda Scott, who was Dr. Riordan's secretary both in private practice and at the origins of The Center, made the transition to the new world well, and coordinated The Center's first International Conference. She knew the man well, and it was doubtless important that there was that continuity close to him.[17]

By the fall of 1976, Dr. Dale Peters also was associated with Dr. Riordan in seeing patients.[18] Dr. Peters, like Dr. Riordan, was outspoken and honest. Once an Associate Professor of Psychiatry at the University of Oklahoma, he had worked for the Sunflower Guidance Center in Concordia, Kansas, and there had contact with Riordan. But he was the first to say he had not always been a supporter of The Center's methods or of its founder. The change came, as so often happens, through a personal experience. Peters's wife was ill, it was found she had low blood sugar, and he was able to observe in her case how much difference a change in diet made in what had seemed intractable problems. He called Riordan, and the two had lunch at a then-popular Wichita restaurant called, rather appropriately given the subject of the meeting, Dr. Redbird's. "The first thing I want to tell you, Riordan," Peters said at that lunch, "is that I have badmouthed you for years, but I have learned I was wrong." Peters was not sure The Center would succeed financially. In fact he eventually left to go into practice in Oklahoma because he felt it could not succeed as a business. Later

---

15 Ibid, July 21, 1980.
16 Interview Laura Benson with Craig Miner, Aug 13, 1999.
17 Ibid.
18 "Throwing A Rope," n.d. c. Oct 1, 1976, CIHF Archives. Hereafter cited as *Rope*.

he admitted he would have to eat those words. But from the time of that early luncheon, he was sure that it could and would succeed in a different way. So in October 1976, he became a part of it. At the first meeting of the psychiatric section at St. Francis Hospital after Peters joined The Center, the section chairman asked Dr. Peters if he wanted to say anything to the group. What he said was unforgettable: "I want you to know that I was an honest fraud like you fellows for years." He had changed his mind, but not his style. His statement may not have helped The Center's physician public relations much, but it demonstrated commitment.[19] "As a result of new leanings partially triggered by personal health experience," the *Rope* announced, "Dale has shifted from his previous strong Freudian orientation to one which encompasses the developing field of Clinical Ecology."[20]

Another member of the early team was Marvin Dirks. Dirks and Riordan met at a Wichita Biofeedback Society meeting and talked in December 1977, while Dirks was working at Prairie View. His broad interests seemed ideal. Dirks's father was a college and seminary professor and his mother a secondary education teacher. The family had traveled widely, living in China and the Philippines beginning in 1939. Dirks played cello and piano, combined a BA from Bluffton College with a BD in theology from Mennonite Seminary in Elkhardt, Indiana, and an MA in psychology from Wichita State University, and had an ongoing interest in comparative religion, international relations, psychophysiology, and airplanes.[21] Still, Riordan had some doubts about hiring him because robbing Prairie View of an employee might not help the good relations The Center had enjoyed with it, and because of the expected abuse that would be directed at The Center and its employees. "We shall most likely be going through a rather difficult period of claims and some restlessness among area psychiatrists concerning our approach to the treatment of 'mental illness.' Although Mr. Dirks has

---

19 Interview, Dr. Hugh Riordan with Craig Miner, May 20, 1998.
20 Letter, Hugh Riordan to Cramer Reed, Oct. 28, 1998, attached to *Rope* of same date.
21 Staff Profiles, CIHF Archives.

had good training for the onslaught that appears to be gathering just over the horizon (he spent three years in a prison camp as a child in the Philippines during World War II), Doctor Riordan wants to make sure Marv knows what he is getting into." Dirks became a half time consultant at The Center early in 1978, at a fee of $300 a month.[22]

The one staff position that The Center thought it needed, but lacked, was an administrator. Dr. Riordan offered to divert some of his pay for this non-budgeted purpose, noting late in 1976 that "because of the significant work overload that built up during our initial months and because of our anticipated growth, an administrator is becoming more essential."[23] Eventually The Center found an effective long-term administrator in Laura Benson, who joined The Center in 1976 part-time to work with the bookkeeping and insurance files. She often backed up other temporary administrators, and observed Riordan's often adding the administrator role to his own work load.[24] She became administrator in 1987 when she told Riordan that it was time to stop the revolving door of administrators.[25] It was difficult to find a person with the careful conservative temperament required for a good accountant and administrator who was suited for the pace of change and the level of risk associated with The Center, particularly in its early years. In November 1976, The Center's bank balance was $7,044.82. It had accounts receivable of $56,855.61. Grants for the year were $142,000, and patient fees of $28,619.32.[26]

Certification of the lab was a top priority. First to come was from the Communicable Disease Center in Atlanta although that proved "elusive" for a time. But Riordan was impressed by the thoroughness of the CDC inspection team that visited in October 1976 and felt that the tougher the standard applied, the more credibility The Center lab would have in doing work for other doctors locally and nationally, and thus helping support financially the research and education missions

---

22 *Rope*, Jan. 3, 1978. Interview, Hugh Riordan with Craig Miner, May 27, 1998.
23 *Rope*, n.d. [c. Oct. 1, 1976].
24 Staff Profiles notebook, CIHF Archives.
25 Interview, Dr. Hugh Riordan with Craig Miner, October 22, 1998.
26 *Rope*, Nov. 1, 1976.

of the organization. It was thought also that this certification, and that by the State of Kansas which came later, would insure that Medicare, Medicaid and private insurance company payments would come automatically to The Center for treatment and lab work.[27]

There were early attempts to attract others to the staff, the most prominent being Dr. Cramer Reed. Reed was a Wichita urologist who was instrumental in establishing both the College of Health Related Professions at Wichita State University and the Wichita Branch of the University of Kansas Medical School, and Riordan knew that he had strong sympathy with the kind of medicine that The Center was advancing.

Riordan approached Reed in the fall of 1976 about associating himself with The Center, or The Center's associating itself with the medical school, or both. Reed seriously considered both, but both, while not out of line with his own inclinations, were too much at variance for the moment with the thinking of too many others. Riordan was more daring, as he had already put his own reputation on the line. He thought that since there was no Department of Clinical Nutrition at any medical school, it would be a source of pride for Wichita to have the first one in the nation "if there is any desire to eventually provide a significant leadership role on the advancing frontiers of medical treatment."[28]

In 1979 Riordan asked Garvey for funding to hire Reed as Director of Health Related Programs with support staff.[29] Reed, however, turned down the opportunity, though he remained a friend and supporter of The Center.[30]

What was clear — from the courting of Reed and the medical school, as well as Riordan's continued activity with the local hospitals, retention of his membership in the Sedgwick County Medical Society, the Kansas Medical Society, and the expensive membership in the American Medical Association, joint grant applications with universi-

---

27 Ibid, Oct. 1, 28, 1976.
28 Dr. Hugh Riordan to Dr. Cramer Reed, Oct 28, 1976 in *Rope*.
29 Letter, Hugh Riordan to Olive Garvey, Oct 24, 1979, Office Files, CIHF Archives.
30 Interview, Dr. Hugh Riordan with Craig Miner, October 22, 1998.

ties and other clinics, as well as numerous speeches to medical groups and attempts, sometimes successful, to publish Center lab results in standard medical journals — was that Dr. Riordan did not wish to be more radical than he had to be.[31] He served as a medical consultant to the Kansas State University guidance center on matters related to nutrition, and interacted with 80 teachers state-wide via the K-State University TV network on the subject of the relationship between nutrition and behavior and intellectual performance.[32]

The Center worked hard and succeeded in having its lab certified with all the regular agencies for accreditation at the state and federal levels. It worked hard, with less success and a considerable feeling of biased treatment, to have care there paid for by medical insurance companies, particularly Blue Cross/Blue Shield. It tried and increasingly did attract to its international conference on Human Functioning in Wichita physicians who would never have described themselves as involved in alternative medicine. And it all the while emphasized that its staff had PhDs and MDs from respected universities.

The employees worked very well together. "It is all too seldom these days," the *Rope* reported late in 1976, "to be able to achieve a closeness between all levels of people showing a common purpose in a common endeavor."[33]

There were many examples of rope throwing by The Center, some more successful than others at making a solid connection. Riordan and Peters provided Dr. David DeJong, the pathologist at St. Francis Hospital and head of its lab, with numerous nutritionally-oriented research works, and, as he absorbed these, The Center's relationship with him grew closer. With DeJong and the University of Kansas, The Center began in

---

31 This insight was reinforced by Laura Benson, The Center administrator, in an interview June 10, 1998. Benson remembered worrying about the cost of the AMA membership, but agreeing with Riordan that it provided reassurance to patients, wanting to try something new, but apprehensive, that he was still a "real" doctor. It took, she said, some really brave patients, to come to The Center in its early years.
32 Ibid, Nov. 15, 1976.
33 *Rope*, Dec. 29, 1976. Interview, Dr. Hugh Riordan with Craig Miner, October 22, 1998.

the fall of 1976 a copper electron spin analysis of selected patients with elevated serum copper levels. One hospitalized patient was given chelation therapy using an amino acid with several chemical "hooks" capable of removing heavy metal ions. This, Riordan reported, "my colleagues severely objected to. Although this patient has had years of unsuccessful psychotherapy, pharmacotherapy and 35 electroshock treatments, these doctors felt I should not be using chelation because it is not universally recognized for treatment of schizophrenia." Riordan offered to have Dr. Pfeiffer appear before the hospital's psychiatric section to discuss his research and clinical observations of the relationship between copper and schizophrenia, but there was no response from the local physicians. "The whole matter," he laconically noted, "will probably go before the research committee of the hospital which is comprised of delightful people who know little about the subjects under discussion.… Thus, as I anticipated, the colleagues are beginning to swoop down and demonstrate their anxiety levels under the guise of concern for patient care." However, not all was dark even there. Dr. DeJong approved of chelation and said he would ask to serve on hospital committees controlling policy.

Slowly other connections were made, and there were small breakthroughs. Thanks to DeJong the lab at St. Francis farmed out certain histamine and kryptopyrrole studies to the lab at The Center, partly because The Center offered to do them for 70% of its usual charge if the hospital would handle the sample collection and billings.[34] Dr. Peters in November 1976 spoke to naturopathic students about some of The Center's work and attended a dinner with them, though "this kind of activity tends to be frowned on by those of our colleagues who prefer not to have an interchange between helping professions." At that time also Riordan was "repeatedly" meeting with the psychiatric section of St. Francis Hospital to discuss the biophysiologic approach to mental illness.[35] At a November 15 meeting with the research committee at the hospital, Riordan agreed to develop protocols for diagnosis and treatment of the various schizophrenias as they were categorized

---

34 *Rope*, Oct. 25, 1976.
35 Ibid, Nov. 15, 1976.

and treated by him and Peters. After four chelations of Riordan's high-copper patient, the young man looked and behaved better than his parents had seen him for years. However, the treatment was once interrupted, and during that time "the patient had to be returned to the locked section of the hospital where he subsequently kicked out a window, crushed a light bulb in his hand, and required frequent use of restraints." However frustrating the experience had been, Riordan thought it was a good demonstration. "These reproducible results are rather encouraging." It was at that time that the mental health center at Prairie View began referring patients to The Center.

Riordan and Peters were themselves encouraged. Riordan reduced his consulting commitment to the Sunflower Guidance Center in Concordia to one long day a month, thus reducing his income. Dr. Peters at the same time phased out his relationship with the Southeast Kansas Mental Health Center in order to devote more time and energy to The Center for the Improvement of Human Functioning.[36] In February of 1977 the two reported that as a result of "patience and friendly cooperation," it would be possible henceforth to administer to patients at St. Francis 12.5 grams of vitamin C in the form of sodium ascorbate intravenously. "This is not being done on a 'research' basis but as therapy recognized by the hospital pharmacy as a developing need at least for the patients of Doctors Peters and Riordan."[37]

DeJong and Riordan began to have regular in-depth discussions of lab procedures with Dr. Charles Hinshaw. The first was of a procedure for detecting kryptopyrrole in the urine. This was a substance Pfeiffer thought robbed the body of zinc and B6 when a metabolic error was present which increased kryptopyrrole excretion. Sometimes in tests it was not this that was detected, but a related pyrrole, porphyryn, which was also a mark of a metabolic disease with many psychiatric symptoms. DeJong's research indicated that rats fed kryptopyrrole developed significant brain wave abnormalities. Perhaps that was why certain epileptics benefited from high doses of vitamin B6. Another discussion related to

---

36 Ibid, n.d. [Nov., 1976].
37 Ibid, Feb. 14, 1977.

some new pH measuring devices (for measuring acidity or alkilinity) being evaluated at The Center. In large "double blind" studies, error could be introduced by the type of water used due the variation in pH between different sorts of water. Perhaps there were no such things as a "blind" treatment or placebo. "No matter what the substance, it will alter the oral pH and subsequently the body chemistry." The more minute the change, the more the placebo would approach a homeopathic type of treatment, which sometimes could have considerable effect. None of Riordan's hospitalized patients had a normal oral pH, as they tended toward the acidic. That seemed worthy of study. The *Rope* reported of these lab talks: "I wish there was some way to convey the very high level of excitement shared by the doctors in relation to the work of The Center and its potential for benefiting mankind. It is a real pleasure for Doctor Riordan to be able to be associated with the two clinical pathologists whose excitement increases as they become more convinced of the biochemical basis of mental and emotional disorders."[38]

But there were bad days. In March 1977 Riordan spoke at a conference on schizophrenia in New York City. He spent 17 hours with leaders in the field and heard "a wealth of derogatory remarks." They laughed at the idea that urine could tell something about schizophrenia, and his frustration rose at the cases he saw who were not being helped. He wanted once, he wrote, "to jump up and scream that the mother of the family was obviously a food sensitive schizophrenic. She had huge dark circles under her eyes ('allergy shiners') and a very puffy face." But the audience just applauded the therapist who was verbally abusing the father in the family. "What is extremely frustrating," Riordan wrote at that time, "is that there are so many people from all over the country who believe that schizophrenia comes only from schizophrenic others." It was a kind of self-perpetuating idea.[39] Riordan often recalled the time when as a student at Wisconsin he had heard a prominent expert on autism give as his explanation for the disease that the mothers of these children were cold and frigid.[40]

---

38 Ibid, n.d. [c. Dec. 1, 1976].
39 Ibid, March 11, 1977.
40 Interview, Dr. Hugh Riordan with Craig Miner, October 22, 1998.

The lab worked on food sensitivities. During 1976 it learned that the top ten were: 1) coffee 2) chocolate 3) cornstarch 4) soybean 5) tobacco 6) egg yolk 7) white potato 8) corn 9) egg white 10) oats. There were studies too of the correlation between CPK levels (an enzyme) and schizophrenic behavior, cytotoxic reactions and emotional disturbances, impaired trace mineral metabolism and depressive and/or schizophrenic behavior, and chronic fatigue, depression and psychosomatic states with altered plasma amino acid patterns. The Center applied for a grant from the American Cancer Society to study the correlation between cytotoxic factors and lung cancer, but since that Society was on record as saying that nutrition had nothing to do with cancer, funding from that source was denied.[41]

Sometimes there was a bright moment in communication. In the spring of 1977 Riordan got a call from Dr. George Dyck, chair of the Department of Psychiatry at the Wichita State University Branch of the University of Kansas School of Medicine. The two had lunch and Dyke brought along a resident named Hart, who had been a chemist and who thought that medicine had gone as far as possible with psychotherapy in depression and schizophrenia. "He believes that all real cures are biochemical and that much research needs to be done in the area of brain biochemistry." He said, "We are thirty years behind in the study of brain biochemistry because the analysts have controlled research funding for that long." Riordan was pleased at the meeting, commenting that "ordinarily such people are kept far from such contact." He took Hart on a tour of The Center's lab, about which Hart "absolutely raved."[42] And there were others around the country of like mind. Riordan commented when he went to a medical conference in Princeton, New Jersey, that Dr. Derrick Lonsdale, a pediatrician doing research in amino acid and vitamin B1 deficiencies would "easily blow the minds of the physicians in attendance who are not yet aware of the enormous significance of vitamins when they are needed."[43]

---

41 *Rope*, April 5, 1977.
42 Ibid, April 18, 1977.
43 Ibid, May 9, 1977.

Certainly Riordan was not one to give up trying to reach the medical profession with his message just because of some rebuffs. In May 1977 he sent a letter to mental health centers around the country. "If you went to medical school anywhere near the time I did (20 plus years ago)," he wrote, "you were not taught about any of the testing procedures which we now believe to be signficiant in the evaluation of those human beings who suffer from unresponsive psychiatric or psychosomatic disorders. Similarly, there is little likelihood that you would have had the opportunity to personally become familiar with the concepts that are involved in the biochemical evaluation of nervous and mental disorders." He himself was skeptical, Riordan wrote, before personal experience taught him otherwise. "For this reason I must assume that you too would be skeptical." But data he included showed that 35% of those patients with "impaired life adjustments" demonstrated elevated urinary pyrrole levels. "The level of urinary pyrrole in these predisposed individuals appears to be directly related to the amount of stress or distress they are experiencing." The Center made available to professionals kits for testing, which they could mail back and for $10 receive an evaluation.[44]

In October there was a letter from Bernard Rimland, PhD, the director of the applied psychobiology program at the Department of the Navy research and development center in San Diego. He had heard about The Center and promised to pay a visit. He hoped, he said, to interest the Navy in orthomolecular/psychobiological approaches to health. "In the past such work has largely fallen in the province of the medical people who are far more interested in worrying about disease than they are in facilitating the positive performance of well personnel."[45]

Orthomolecular medicine, defined as using substances that normally occur in the body that are not toxic to the body to combat disease at a cellular level, was a key element of The Center's approach. The phrase was originated by Dr. Linus Pauling, who co-authored a book about it. So significant did The Center's work become to the whole field that in

---
44 Ibid, May 11, 1977.
45 Letter, Rimland to Riordan, Oct. 26, 1977, in *Rope*.

the late 1990s the *Journal of Orthomolecular Medcine* contained each quarter an article called "Cases from The Center," which detailed the stories of patients helped in Wichita by that approach.[46]

And so there were these contacts, here and there, near and far, and attempts to define The Center *vis a vis* others. Meanwhile, Riordan kept studying himself. He tried a 14 day distilled water and lemon juice fast, but had to abandon it early when his uric acid level rose sufficiently for him to be concerned about gout.[47] Dr. Peters at the same time was taking 45 grams of vitamin C a day "without any evidence of uncorking."[48]

Patients benefited from a different approach in Wichita. One young woman came to a mental health center where Riordan was a consultant. She could not attend high school because of her mental illness. She had white spots on her fingernails and knee pain, classic physical symptoms for which Pfeiffer always looked. She was taken off her medicines, put on vitamin therapy, and in a couple of weeks was totally normal. Before she and her family would believe it was so simple, however, she went off the vitamin regimen and regressed four times. Eventually, however, she stuck with Riordan's recommendation and became state champion baton twirler and a straight A student. She later married, had children, and had no further psychiatric problems.

Could it be proven in a large double blind study that this vitamin treatment was effective? No. For one thing it worked on only about 20% of schizophrenics, which would be below the level of the placebo effect in such a study, and, second, there was no funding for such a large study. So stories like the baton twirler's cure were "anecdotal" and as such were dismissed by many physicians. But it was what The Center people began to call an "N of one" study. That the person helped was only one individual did not make their cure a bit less certain. Double blind studies were originally based on agricultural research, which was concerned with the field or the herd and not with how one cow or wheat plant was doing. There was also the agricultural assumption of

---

46 Interview, Dr. James Jackson with Craig Miner, Sept. 10, 1999.
47 *Rope*, June 15, 1977.
48 Ibid, Aug. 1, 1977.

homogeneity of "product," something that was perhaps inapplicable and probably inappropriate to human beings. Riordan himself dismissed some of the criticism that people improved when they came to The Center because they were desperate, knew it was their last chance, and therefore, in effect healed themselves. If so, he said, that was fine with him. The focus should be on the result, not the process, and not where the credit lay. Even so-called placebo effects might be tapping some deep and important healing resource in the human organism, and so-called psychosomatic illnesses might well be a more subtle variation of a standard illness.

While there were questions by some doctors about how useful the tests done by the new Center lab were, most were impressed that such information as it could provide could be made available at all. Particularly interesting was the capability of building a fairly complete biochemical profile of an individual by integrating various tests, some of which had been done before in isolation, and some of which had not been done at all. If the patient were to be treated as an individual, unique and separate from other individuals, but at the same time as a cohesive and interdependent single entity internally, the standard approaches had to be turned on their heads. Therefore the techniques and lab tests of many specialists, from allergists to psychiatrists, were combined at The Center and considered simultaneously in diagnosis. In a way the assumptions went back to an axiom of ancient Greek medicine that health was a kind of balance, and that an imbalance anywhere in the body could have a chain of effects that reached as far from its source as that mysterious noise in somebody's car. Why should lack of B-vitamins lead to depression and a black tongue, both hallucination and sore knees? Why should exercise produce endorphins that lead to a feeling of well-being? Could cancer be triggered by stress? One did not have to understand fully the answer to those questions to grasp the links and follow the chains.

A lot of what the lab did, said Riordan, "many doctors don't even know you can do." The response of some doctors was watchful waiting and respectful interest. Others were contemptuous. Still others were quiet at first in the certainty that "we would go away" and then more aggressive as it became clear that The Center was surviving, even growing.[49]

Case studies mounted, and they were not the spoiled hypochondriac type, but people so seriously ill that others had given up on them. And the thickness of the file of appreciative letters grew. There was a 15-year-old boy who was aggressive and destructive, had white spots on his fingernails and ate chocolate candy with a passion. There was a 24-year-old woman, daughter of a CPA, who was so withdrawn she seldom went outside the house, and whose fantasy life was her only joy. "Although she expressed the feeling that she could never stand to have anyone touch her, especially a man, Doctor Riordan held her hand throughout the initial interview." She sobbed that day, something she had never been able to do. Lab tests showed she was anemic with very low iron and strong food sensitivities. Her mother had had a nervous breakdown a few years earlier and a brother had committed suicide. A 26-year-old man came in, almost completely immobile. He needed help even to take off his glasses. He had diabetes and sub scurvy plasma levels of vitamin C. There was a 30-year-old minister who had had to give up church because of tiredness, depression, a slow heart beat and numbness. He was sensitive to sugar. A 23-year-old male patient had tried to kill himself three times, the third attempt by hanging, before he saw Dr. Riordan. His father read Dr. Pfeiffer's book in The Center's waiting room and suggested that his son was suffering from "Sarah's syndrome." That was perceptive. "There is a strong likelihood," Riordan wrote, "that his mother and other family members have been burdened with inborn errors of metabolism which contributed significantly to their mental illness." Before the end of that first interview this young man was able to manage a small smile and to shake Riordan's hand. Eventually he went to a university in California without any medication.[50]

About the same time Riordan saw a man who was catatonic. It took five minutes to get him to stand from a seated position. He had withdrawn from law school and been repeatedly hospitalized over four

---

49 Interview, Dr. Hugh Riordan with Craig Miner, May 27, 1998.
50 *Rope*, Aug. 8, 1977.

years. The Center found he had low vitamin C and zinc. After receiving these intravenously and orally he began to feel better than at any time in his adult life, and he was able to go back to law school.[51]

That was rewarding. Wrote one patient: "I'm fine.... I am even brave and fine now. I got out the journal I kept before coming to The Center and almost couldn't believe the agony expressed on those pages. I stopped writing the journal after coming to The Center because I got involved in getting better."[52] Another returned to The Center in 1978, two years after his initial treatment, both to thank the people there and to ask for advice on nutrition in his career as a straight A pre-med student. Riordan's comment was that; "The change in this young man in two years from 'I have no memory — I read and forget immediately — I'm talking and my mind goes blank and nothing is there — my concentration is very bad' to being able to maintain straight As in a tough program is just another example of how important nutrients such as he was lacking can be." He contacted Mrs. Garvey to thank her for her vision in supporting The Center.[53] The *Rope* reported, "Although somewhat exhausting, it is a real thrill for Doctor Riordan to be able to see and provide hope for human beings who previously considered themselves hopeless."[54]

Diagnosis and treatment at The Center shortly began to move beyond the purely psychological to psychosomatic and chronic metabolic illnesses. Perhaps as a preparation, Riordan in November of 1976 began one of his famous self studies, using his own body for some 200 days of lab studies which included days of normal diet, fasting and special vitamin and mineral intakes, with frequent tests.[55] He found a variety of foods that caused his heart to skip beats and early in 1977 he was able to produce multiple joint pains with a high sugar diet and then to reduce them by simultaneous ingestion of high levels of vita-

---

51 Ibid, Nov. 14, 1977.
52 Ibid, Sept. 19, 1977.
53 Ibid, Aug. 28, 1978.
54 Ibid, Aug. 8, 1977.
55 Ibid, n.d. [Nov., 1976].

min C.[56] Shortly, lessons began to be applied to patients other than those suffering from mental illnesses.

There was great success, on the order of 90%, with migraine headaches. The Center did blood histamine level tests, having found either too high or too low levels of this neurotransmitter could trigger headaches.

Migraines and enormously painful cluster headaches were also treated successfully with large doses of vitamin C (several grams a day, sometimes given intravenously). Intravenous C could in many patients stop a cluster headache in progress before the patient was out of the office. Given how debilitating these were and how relatively simple and inexpensive the treatment, those getting relief became convinced supporters of The Center and its approach.

Adverse food reactions were another migraine culprit. Riordan himself once had migraines, and found that they could be relieved by eating chocolate. Then he found that in fact chocolate was the cause as well as, ironically, the temporary cure, and by avoiding it he avoided headaches.

In order to reduce the time, frustration, and complications involved in the trial and error method of testing food reactions by simply withdrawing a food, The Center began doing food allergy tests involving the reaction of a person's own white cells. These tests, pioneered by George Ulett, MD, PhD and allergist William Bryan, MD were and remain among the most controversial tests that The Center does. However, in migraines and other ailments it seemed clear to the doctors there that food sensitivities mattered, and that white cells were "little brains" that responded to neurochemicals as the whole body would respond to these substances in food. There were also some signs which were tip-offs, including dark circles around the eyes. These allergic shiners often suggest underlying food sensitivities.

Actually, everyday observation establishes the centrality of food sensitivities. Dr. Riordan joked in his talks on gas and bloating (something few physicians talk about at luncheon meetings and about which everyone is afraid to ask) that any trucker knows that when you eat beans you have a reaction. Every physician knows that serotonin has

---

56 Ibid, Feb. 14, 1977.

something to do with the way you feel mentally, and drugs like Prozac are largely serotonin sparers, and if a doctor orders a lab test to measure serotonin, the patient is told that for 72 hours he or she should not eat certain foods because they either raise or lower serotonin. Physicians have known for centuries that certain diseases are nutritional deficiencies: scurvy, pellagra and Beri-Beri, for example. Yet applying that more broadly has been a slow process.

How one ate as well as what one ate was important. Dr. Riordan tested many things on himself— in fact most things. He rarely used a procedure or a substance on a patient that he had not tried personally. He did not get a headache every time he ate chocolate. It might depend on whether he was eating in "serene" or stressful circumstances. And it might depend on the rest of his diet, or his exercise program, or how his life or work generally was going. So it was with others. A person who was a pyrrole excreter and tended to lose B6 and zinc in urine might have few problems if she ate vegetables while praying, but considerable difficulty if eating meat during business meetings. B6 is necessary to digest animal protein.

The pace of eating in the US had accelerated. Fast food places apologized for making people wait more than 30 seconds for their food, and those customers often spent only 30 seconds wolfing it down. The kind and variety of foods available had changed. Once Canada shipped twenty different kinds of apples to the US, but that was reduced to the six that packed and lasted best. Having fewer kinds of food generated more food reactions in people who were susceptible, just as Dutch Elm Disease thrives where there are only elms. There were a large number of considerations in food sold other than nutritional value or natural flavor. Yet every change and every choice affected bodies that were not evolving nearly as fast as the switch to processed food marketing. Even "health" foods could be quite artificial, and there were regular debates about the safety of artificial sweeteners and the meaning of "low fat." People were understandably confused when they were told one day that bran was the answer, the next that it was a fad; that cholesterol was the villain, then that it was not; that vitamins were great, or could be toxic; that there were many kinds of fat and you needed some of all of them; that it was hormone balance not supply of a single hormone that mattered; or that suddenly, alcohol consumption in moderation was OK. Fad diets were healthy primarily for the bank accounts of their publishers and authors.

Consequently The Center recognized early that the nutritional regimen it hoped would eventually prevail would require considerable public education. That was the reason for beginning its series of international conferences, its book and newsletter publication program, and its audio and video taped luncheon lectures. For nutrition as an answer was simple in one way and complex in another. It was "natural," but hardly instinctual in modern society. Try to find alfalfa to eat as an antioxidant or sea kelp as an iodine source or fish oil for essential fatty acids, and then try to eat those in the quantities recommended. And it was not just the level of a nutrient that one was taking in, but how the body metabolized it, even the speed at which the body metabolized and excreted it, that really mattered. One of Riordan's trials on himself was to take one 500 mg. tablet of panothenic acid, a B vitamin, after fasting for three days. "I thought I was going to die. My legs felt like they were lead." Fat was liberated and his triglycerides went out of sight, yet he had simply taken a natural substance under certain circumstances. The whole business of using nature to regulate health took a lot more knowledge, responsibility, and discipline than swallowing a pill.

Yet the direction was so promising it seemed worth it. One can turn a huge ocean-going ship with a tiny rudder, Riordan has said. "If you wanted to change the health of the country in a year, the government should give everyone a small herb garden." In his opinion the effect of having fresh, unprocessed foods available —"something that from the time it was harvested to the time it went into your mouth was only a few minutes" — would be enormous.

Rheumatoid arthritis responded to The Center's testing and the nutritional therapy. The first person treated there for rheumatoid arthritis was Marge Page, the wife of Bob Page, Mrs. Garvey's chief business advisor. As with treating Mrs. Garvey herself, this case was a bit frightening, as Dr. Riordan knew that Page was "verbal" and would spread the word about The Center, positive or negative. But she needed help. She was a musician who could not play the piano because of her illness and a golfer who had not been able to hold her clubs for about a year, in spite of standard medical treatment. Bio Center Lab tests revealed several things. First, she was sensitive to corn. Not eating corn by itself was easy, but then one had to learn what products contained corn. One of them was beer. Page called every manufacturer to learn that the only domestic beer made without corn at that time was Michelob. She switched to that. She was a smoker and had a high lead level, so began chelation at The Center to remove that. The result was that her arthritis eased and she was able again to do all the things she had been forced to forgo. She was back to playing golf in three weeks. And, as was the pattern with people who were helped there, the Pages became not only verbal, but financial supporters of The Center, among the first major donors after Mrs. Garvey herself. And Marge Page was a good example of a co-learner. The Center's goal is to convert patients to co-learners who become very knowledgeable about how to improve their health.

Clearly, too, the incidental involvement of Marge's husband Bob in this experience, had important later ramifications for The Center. Bob Page was the major business and financial advisor to the Garvey family, as well as to other families and corporations around the United States, was a CPA as well as an attorney, and was well-recognized for his genius and judgment. In his role with Mrs. Garvey, he automatically had been involved in The Center's affairs, but his wife's near miraculous recovery as a result of treatment there gave him a personal example that was irreplaceable in generating a personal enthusiasm for its mission. It was to be Mr. Page who in future years was instrumental in helping The Center become financially self-supporting, and he was always ready to mentor its people in the fiscal disciplines of which he was a master.

Treating arthritis as a food sensitivity or by looking for infection — the whole idea that there was an underlying cause for it that could be treated — was controversial in the early years. "When you went to a rheumatologist," Riordan recalled, "they were going to teach you to live with the disease. I thought it would be more appropriate to go to a priest, or a boy scout or a minister if that's what you were going to do."

Other ailments responded too, not to standard, but to customized treatment, but all based on the same assumptions about the complex effects of nutritional deficiencies in people with individual biochemistry. Depression could be caused by all sorts of things. One of them was low vitamin C. That had been known in the literature for many years, and Riordan could not understand why psychiatrists did not regularly test depression patients for Vitamin C level in the blood. Earlier The Center did studies with patients at the nearby Prairie View mental health facility and at St. Francis Hospital and found that about one-third of the patients admitted for depression were low in vitamin C. But there were other causes. An early client was a woman from Michigan, who still wrote to The Center 25 years later, whose son at age eight was suicidal, and when in school would go to the candy store, eat candy and sob. Through diagnosis and treatment, The Center helped him, and mother and son became believers in The Center's approach.

Probably vitamin C is the most used treatment at The Center: it was in the 1990s given to slow cancer and increase quality of life in terminal patients. As usual, Riordan used his own therapy and took 200 *grams* of vitamin C intravenously a couple of times with no ill effects. Once he was bitten by a spider just at the time for his monthly C level test. The test showed his vitamin C level was undetectable. He took 15 grams intravenously, and it was still undetectable. On the fifth day after the bite, it got into the scurvy range before massive doses brought it back up. It did not come up until the spider bite began to heal. This experience was a real turning point in his life. He really understood the connection between a toxin and vitamin C plasma levels. Just how much C it requires to overcome something like a spider bite was amazing to him.

High blood pressure is often called "essential hypertension." This means that the cause is unknown. But The Center saw little essential about it or the usual treatments for it. People with high blood pressure were not being told what the cause of it was, just to "take this medicine for the rest of your life and all will be fine." The Center tried chelation.

That was something that raised hackles, but helped patients. Riordan noted that when he first started using chelation "it was not controversial at all because it was not interfering with the cottage industry of cardiovascular surgery." But it became controversial, so much so that there was an attempt by the Board of Healing Arts to outlaw it in Kansas. Chelation, using an amino acid complex whose molecules remove ions of heavy metals, was originally invented to treat lead poisoning. The US government reportedly has large stockpiles of EDTA, which is the chelation agent, because it is the only thing that will save people with radiation poisoning. Lead levels seem to correlate with hypertension. Two large studies conducted by The Centers for Disease Control concluded that the strongest correlation with high blood pressure was lead level. The Center had good success with lowering blood pressure because chelation not only removed lead, but allowed blood vessels to dilate. Lead has been much implicated in reducing IQ in children especially. Chelation can be used to remove other heavy metals also, which are an increased risk in the modern environment. That, combined with the effect in dilating the blood vessels, is the reason for its application in high blood pressure and cardiovascular disease generally. In some countries, governments actually pay for chelation.

Again by supporting this controversial treatment and applying it successfully to individuals, friends were made for The Center over the years. Richard Lewis, who was first employed by The Center as Director of Development in 1985 and later edited the *Health Hunter* newsletter, tested at a biological age (determined by a series of physical tests) of more than 15 years less than his actual age and gave most convincing tours to visitors, had been in a series of industrial jobs and was taking three hypertension medicines when he arrived. After a series of chelations, he had no "essential" hypertension or in fact high blood pressure at all. Such a personal health care program beyond the usual insurance plan is one reason Center staff has little turnover and the service pins for five or more years are common. That pin, incidentally, contains a pearl for each five years served. The pearl symbolizes The Center, which once seemed an irritant and became a thing of beauty. The development brochure for The Center in the 21st century was entitled "The Pearl" to reflect this symbolism.

Something vaguely called "irritable bowel syndrome" was a chronic problem for many, and one which was often both an embarrassing and fruitless topic of inquiry. Operations for bowel problems such as Crohn's disease were costly and often ineffective, and the cure might be as simple as ridding the bowel of a parasite, or eating differently. Parasite treatment in the 1990s became a specialty of The Center, so much so that it patented a new way of looking for some parasites. The pertinent question that Center doctors would ask was: "Why does it make sense to the body and the bowel? There is no reason to say 'I have a stupid bowel' and cut it out. That doesn't make any sense."

These were new approaches to well-known ailments, but The Center also studied things that some were not sure were real — such as Extra Sensory Perception. Susan Cottrell, who moved to Wichita in 1976, had remarkable powers of this type, and The Center tried to study her so as to document the source of her ability, for example, to predict what card a person would pick from a pack and cause them to do it.[57] She did this accurately even with a babe in arms who simply grabbed for the cards with obviously no forethought whatsoever.[58] The national press picked up the story in 1977 and did interviews with her and with Dr. Riordan. "Let's hope, " Riordan wrote, "they don't distort the story too badly."[59] Later she was on the Johnny Carson show.

The Center, through use of biofeedback, obtained some hard data regarding Cottrell's ESP ability. Riordan wrote that "this is, to my knowledge, the first time something like this has ever been accomplished in the world."[60] People were seated around a table and with heat sensors on their fingers attached to a meter. They could not see their meter or anyone else's. With the cards all face down, a card was mentally selected by Miss Cottrell as the one for a person to choose. She would select the Queen of Hearts, for example, and the person would choose from the entire deck. When the subject touched the face down card, his or her finger tip temperature went up significantly (and

---

57 Ibid, Dec. 6, 1976.
58 Interview, Dr. Hugh Riordan with Craig Miner, June 10, 1998.
59 *Rope*, Feb. 14, 1977.
60 Letter, Hugh Riordan to Paul Black, NBC Tonight Show, Feb. 21, 1977 in *Rope*, March 1, 1977. See also *Rope*, March 11, 1977.

when observing to a lesser extent). She said at a demonstration at the Department of Psychology at Kansas State University that she could make even an infant pick an ace, but she wanted to have four tries. So the entire deck was presented to the infant, who was held in the father's arms, and the infant simply touched cards and in four times picked four aces. However, ensuing complications in trying to study Cottrell ended the investigation.[61]

Riordan came to call this sort of phenomena "subtle energies." His approach was that of a scientist, looking for a physical basis for that kind of communication. And it personalized a phenomenon that might have otherwise seemed remote and unlikely.

Dr. Riordan himself had a strange but important experience in unexplained communication at about that same time. He owned a Cessna 210, which he loaned to other physicians regularly. One Sunday morning as he was in his office ready to leave for the hospital, he got a very strong mental message to call a woman whom he knew, but with whom he did not regularly communicate. He called and there was no answer. Later, about to leave again, he had another strong feeling that this woman needed him. He called again, got no answer and went to the hospital. A half hour later he received a call from a dentist friend that another dentist had borrowed Riordan's plane. As he later learned, that dentist was preparing for take off with the woman in question in the passenger seat. Apparently he had left the ignition on, which resulted in a dead battery, so he was hand cranking the propeller with the woman sitting inside. The engine started and the plane actually took off. The second mental message Riordan had gotten was at 8:15. The woman, who had no knowledge of flying, had been helpless in the air 400 miles away in Arkansas at precisely that time. At 8:18 the plane had crashed and she was killed. "This was an amazing thing to me," Riordan recalled years later, understating the case.

Riordan had friends who would have tried to explain to him how this communication could have happened. When discussing the situation with researcher Dr. Phil Callahan, he said that the answer was

---

61 Interview, Dr. Hugh Riordan with Craig Miner, June 10, 1998.

quite simple, that the atmosphere was like a florescent tube and if two people were tuned to the same frequency, a message could get through. But Riordan did not have to understand it to believe it. "That experience really changed my perception." Because the plane was underinsured and the Internal Revenue Service thought the insurance claim was a financial windfall, it was the end of Riordan's flying his own plane. But it was the beginning of his taking ESP very seriously. "I wish I had known what she wanted," he said, "I would have told her how to land the plane." He went to the woman's grave waiting for another message, but none ever came. Still, to him it was an example of his own maxim that "once you know, it is impossible to not know. And you are forever changed."[62]

Some investigations were a bit closer to the mainstream, but still unusual. Riordan, for example, personally had a sensitivity to fluorescent lights, and felt that office lighting, particularly of the cheaper variety, could cause workers health problems. Dr. Richard Guthrie, chair of the Department of Pediatrics at the University of Kansas Medical School branch in Wichita had a related interest in the effects of the use of narrow band blue light for treatment of jaundice in newborns, and Riordan, Guthrie and Dr. Vic Eichler of the Department of Biology at Wichita State University had some discussions of that in 1977. Drs. Riordan and Eichler visited the General Electric Lighting Institute in Cleveland and also Massachusetts Institute of Technology to meet with those who had researched the effects of lighting on people.[63]

Typically, The Center tried right away to apply the theories about light to the problems of patients. One of them was a lady from Oklahoma who was going blind despite the efforts of seven ophthalmologists. She had a rare type of uveitis, they said, but they had no idea of the cause. She told them she was bothered by fluorescent lights, but each told her they were the best type. The Center, when she visited it in 1978, took her to its frog growth research lab, where it was testing the effects of different kinds of light on the growth of tadpoles, and asked her to

---

62 Ibid, May 20, 1998.
63 *Rope*, Nov. 14, Dec. 12, 1977.

look at pure spectrum green, red, blue and standard fluorescents. She felt best in the red, the opposite response of most people. Dr. Riordan visited her work place with two other people from The Center and carrying a tape recorder, a magnetometer, an AM radio to measure errant RF or radio frequencies, ultra violet monitoring equipment, and black and white Kirlian photo apparatus.

"What we found," Riordan reported, "was nothing short of amazing." Riordan felt discomfort in her office within 30 minutes. The light above her head produced high frequency radio waves. Kirlian photos of her fingertips showed that the energy flow dramatically changed depending on whether or not the overhead light was on. Members of the research team did not show such changes. "It was as though a switch was turned on in her body when the light over her head was on." She had a large desk top electronic calculator. It sat on her right and she had begun going blind in her right eye. There was a vigorous radio frequency directional signal toward where she sat, which lead screening would stop. Her legs were cold, and she kept a heater under her desk which also produced electromagnetic and radio frequencies. In short, what seemed an innocent enough workplace could be, at least for this woman, fraught with hazard, yet there was nothing which a little investigation and some simple countermeasures could not change. She was in her twenties and the alternative was a lifetime of blindness. Yet, certainly, the doctors poring over her office with all this equipment, must have seemed an odd group to more traditional science. What could lights, a calculator and the growth of frogs have to do with it?[64] Yet when the heater was removed, the calculator was lead lined and one overhead fixture was replaced, her vision stopped deteriorating because she was no longer triangulated by electromagnetic activity.[65]

Another plausible but controversial interest of The Center at this time was longevity. The work of Dr. Johan Bjorksten, Dr. Riordan's former boss in Wisconsin, suggested that life in reasonably good health could be extended possibly to as much as 200 years. While the medical

---

64 Ibid, June, 1978.
65 Interview, Dr. Hugh Riordan with Craig Miner, October 22, 1998.

news in 1998 was quite matter of fact about the imminent possibility of training cells to sustain more divisions and to accomplish just that, it was "off the wall" talk in the 1970s. The Center's library was collecting literature on the powers of substitution of the brain's 12 billion cells and the opportunities in redundant metabolism for lengthening life. One simple possibility was the control of diet. If one never ingested more than the body could process straight through "in minimum time and cleanly," the bottlenecks in the metabolic process represented by enzymes might be broadened. Also, longevity could be increased by the optimal supply of vitamins, all of which had multiple functions. Bjorksten wrote that "the vitamins have been elaborated by organisms over millions of years. It is thus understandable that every time an organism in its evolution encountered a new chemical need, it would first experiment with those powerful chemicals which it already had evolved." The concept of "recommended doses" of vitamins was flawed. Before any overt symptoms of disease appeared, the body had used all its reserves. Last, it was important to avoid poisoning oneself.

Given a plausible human lifetime of 90 years, by then any chemical reaction that was theoretically possible would have actually occurred, and any resulting product from those that was insoluable and irremovable would become life threatening by that age. Ways must be found to prevent the buildups or remove them, and the body was not too good at this, since it was not concerned with survival beyond the reproductive and child-rearing years necessary for the survival of the species. But the "low yield, slow reaction effects" were just what the new medicine must watch most closely. "There is no 'time bomb' or programmed death," Center visitors could read. "The post reproduction deaths which now invariably occur sometime between 50 and 160 years are simply the results of the absence of defense against the innumerable slow reactions." There was no talk of immortality, but the prospect of another 50-70 years, achieved with mostly a little lifestyle discipline, was for a person with something to do in life a prospect as attractive as it was to Center physicians interested in the quality of those lives.[66]

---

66 *Rope*, Nov. 7, 1977.

Olive Garvey, Riordan remembered, was not overly impressed. "That man may be an expert on aging," she commented at a lecture, "but he looks pretty old to me."[67]

These early clinical investigations and patients, humdrum to bizarre, as they moved The Center away from the admittedly profitable business of total focus on referred difficult psychiatric cases to a broader scope of nutritionally-based wellness, created an atmosphere there that was nearer the core values of Riordan and of Garvey. Riordan's sharp sense of humor missed no irony, and one of them is that it is hard to raise money for a non-profit institution by being in the wellness business. It is well known in medical circles that contributions come from the families of the patient who has not survived: that is the area where more research needs to be done, ironically, to correct the mistakes made on the loved one of those funding it.

Wellness, for one thing, seemed so right and so inevitable when health was present that the clinic or physician generally got little or no credit for maintaining it. And even when a "miraculous" cure was effected, the well-educated patient perceived and the alternative physician admitted that it was mostly the power of the body itself that created it. What was less obvious was how much skill and experience it took to get the body working as it should, how vital small changes in lifestyle or diet might be, and how devastating the disease avoided might have been. Those who escape forget, and those who never experience don't vividly imagine.

All the cells in the body, except for those in the brain and spinal cord, are completely replaced in six years. So, in six years it is clearly possible to be entirely a "new person." But, Riordan noticed, "six years is beyond the pale for most people." There is a reluctance to change ingrained habits. A Center patient brought a friend to lunch at The Center who asked whether if she came there she would have to change her diet. Told she undoubtedly would she responded: "I can't do that. I'll just die." Another factor making the new treatment difficult to sustain is that when someone is really cured, he doesn't come back for further

---

67 Interview, Dr. Hugh Riordan with Craig Miner, October 22, 1998.

expensive treatment. Therefore, the goal of a place like The Center for the Improvement of Human Functioning — to get rid of patients by eliminating their ailments — was in a way a conflict of interest.

Still, it was possible to change attitudes and to change minds. It happened slowly, and it didn't happen to everybody, but to those who saw, everything was transformed. Consistently about 30% of The Center's contributions came from its former patients. And it was necessary for Riordan, and in time for the staff he hired, to feel that they were devoting their time and energy to a system that did no harm and was not a revolving door of illness. Many standard treatments in 1975, chemotherapy for cancer among them, would, in Riordan's view be "viewed like bloodletting in fifty years." Yes, they became more sophisticated and more effective, but such treatments were still "pretty much Old Testament. If the part offends you, you get rid of it one way or the other." To Riordan and his growing group it was time "to move on to the New Testament."[68]

The Bio Center Lab, for example, was and remains a state-of-the-art medical laboratory, limited in staff size and funding, but hardly by its expertise or efficiency. Equipment came along with staff. There was an Atomic Absorption Spectrophotometer and an Amino Acid Analyzer, for example, not only to be used, but regularly to be repaired.[69] These could be a problem — as Dr. Yeh put it once as a PS to a report — "All Instruments Must Behave Themself" — but when they behaved there were fine results.[70] Late in 1977 The Center reported average monthly expenditures of a little over $17,000, and Riordan said he wanted enough time free from direct patient care to do public relations and fundraising. The lab needed then: an atomic absorbtion furnace for trace mineral studies, a dual beam stectrophotometer for enzyme studies, photomicroscopy equipment to verify cytotoxic tests, a gastrointestinal pH measuring device, and biofeedback monitoring

---

68 Ibid, Dr. Hugh Riordan with Craig Miner, June 3, 1998.
69 Ibid.
70 *Rope*, Dec 7, 1976.

equipment, to mention just part of the "wish" list.[71]

The Center joined others in applying for grants. In 1976, Ailene Fraiker, PhD, submitted a joint grant application from the University of Kansas Medical School in Wichita and the Institute of Logopedics there to study amino acid patterns in autistic children. The Center's lab was to do 185 of these and receive over $13,000 in funding. That showed respect for the lab's capabilities.

In 1978, as the original period of Garvey funding ended, The Center letterhead listed as divisions: the Bio Center Laboratory, the Nutritional Biochemistry Research Laboratory, the Kirlian Phenomenon Laboratory, the Cytotoxic Evaluation Laboratory, and the Amino Acid Evaluation Laboratory. Peters was Director of Clinical Ecology, Hinshaw, Director of Laboratories, and Yeh, Director of Research. In addition to Dirks, other consultants were Carl Pfeiffer, MD, PhD, and Dr. David DeJong, the pathologist at St. Francis.[72] Two international conferences had been completed. It had been a modest start, but a successful one.

Neither Riordan nor Garvey, however, were of a type to leave it at that. They therefore made the close of the decade a watershed time for The Center. Not only did it move well beyond its original mission and into the broad task of creating an "epidemic of wellness" in the world, but it began to expand its patient base well beyond physician-referred mental cases or even people with what were considered serious illness, and it expanded its education function considerably. Perhaps most dramatically, it planned to move from its non-descript collection of buildings on Oliver and on Douglas streets to a "Master Facility" that in appearance as well as in function would suggest to all who viewed and visited that they were indeed on the cusp of the future.

---

71 Ibid, Nov. 9, 1977.
72 Ibid, Jan. 3, 1978.

Chapter Three
Personal Health Control

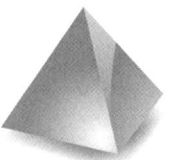

An innovation of the late 1970s that had repercussions far into the future of The Center was the international conference on Human Functioning, first held in September 1977. The Biomedical Synergistics Institute was created at The Center in 1976 to advance the educational program that had to be a feature of its next stage of development. It was a necessary step to advance the educational process among colleagues and the community at large. Also, it would be a step to indicate that The Center would not go away as quickly as some had hoped. There was discussion that fall of bringing to Wichita "the kinds of biomedical minds who are pushing the frontiers of medicine," and establishing for that purpose a liaison with the WSU college of health-related sciences and the Wichita branch of the KU medical school. That far Cramer Reed was willing to go, and students attending The Center's conferences were able to receive college credit, increasing the audience.

The first official function was a visit to Wichita by Dr. Herman Feingold, whose diet for hyperactive children, based on the removal of food colorings and salicylates, was getting publicity and generating controversy. Feingold had dinners with Dr. and Mrs. Cramer Reed, Mr. and Mrs. Cliff Allison, psychologists representing mental health centers in 20 Kansas counties, and medical students, most of the events being held at Wichita State University. He toured The Center. He lectured at Wichita's Century II Convention Center, and again to a neurology class at the Institute of Logopedics and to a group at the medical school. There was no charge for attending, and planning got underway to bring Dr. Carl Pfeiffer for the same kind of local tour.

There were two problems for Riordan. One was that eventually there needed to be a way to charge a fee, as Garvey tended to provide seed money rather than endowments. Second, it was important that the speakers be stimulating, daring, but not offensive. "One of the greatest problems I personally feel pressure about, "Riordan wrote his planners, "is that the biomedical minds we bring in must be on the frontier of medicine and yet not so antagonistic toward status quo medicine that they are turned off by those who need to learn." Pfeiffer had been key in the founding of The Center and would "attract a large lay audience but…might alienate a large segment of those with whom we have already established rapport." Pfeiffer was saying publicly that the government should do away with mental health centers and replace them with Brain Bio Centers. Riordan's response to that was "I feel that our position of educating mental health personnel and challenging our Directors to 'do it our way' for two years on those patients who don't respond is much more tenable."[1]

Both the financial and the public relations concerns were addressed by creating a conference the next year. A conference could be more easily viewed as a balanced educational experience and charged for accordingly. It would involve leading figures in the field with The Center and with Wichita. It would draw larger crowds of persons who would be interested in at least one of the speakers. And any controversy would be less likely to dominate the entire coverage. The catered meals that were served at the conference were much and favorably commented upon and were part of the nutrition education process.

Dr. Riordan studied other conferences. He went to the "New Boundaries for Health" conference in Boston and then to the Society for Orthomolecular Medicine conference in Princeton, New Jersey. At

---

1 Ibid, Oct 4, 1976.

these meetings he networked with others in the field and began to line up a program for the Wichita event.[2]

By June a speaker's list had developed. John Bjorksten PhD would speak on the cross linkage concept in aging; Dr. Everetts Loomis on the clinical benefits of fasting; Dr. Gerald Looney of the University of Southern California School of Medicine on "the greatest untapped health resource" (the patient); Dr. Derrick Lonsdale of the Cleveland Clinic on vitamin B1; Dr. Gladys McGarey of Phoenix on current birthing processes; Dr. William McGarey on holistic treatment; Dr. John Ott on the effects of different wave lengths on the endocrine system; Robert Nunley, PhD, from the University of Kansas, on computerized visualization techniques; Dr. Catherine Spears, a pediatric neurologist who shortly would become a Center consultant, on how B6 and zinc affects behavior and learning stress, and Roger Williams, PhD, of the University of Texas on nutrition generally.[3]

The symbol of that first conference was a complex graphic, chosen after a competition among graphic design students, which was described as a "dendridic representation of the Greek letter psi," and which combined a stylized wheat head with a version of the staff of Aesculapius.[4] Another symbol, which became a bit controversial, was an ostrich saying "My Head's Out of the Sand." The slogan was developed through student competition. Some took offense at the implication that traditional medicine had its head in the sand, and The Center had to send out sheets explaining that was not the intent.[5] It was reported that "about one eight hour segment per day of Doctor Riordan's life will be devoted to the conference until it comes to fruition."[6] How many of these "segments" he managed to put into his style of day was not specified.

Certainly he was excited about the conference. "The incredible line-up of biochemical minds that we are bringing to Wichita for

---

2 *Rope*, May 9, 1977.
3 Ibid, June 6, 1977.
4 Ibid, June 15, 1977.
5 Ibid, Sept. 19, 1977.
6 Ibid, Aug. 1, 1977.

the September conference," he wrote late in August, "should literally shake the foundations of the belief systems of those professionals who have chosen to ignore or who have been unaware of the importance of nutrition and the ramifications in health and disease." Looking at his budget, he understood why nearly every other medical conference was 50% funded by drug companies, but wanted "no vested interest" dominating the agenda at this one. One of the interesting facets of these conferences in the early days was that expenses were paid, but no faculty member was paid for his or her presentation because the participation by the distinguished faculty was based on relationships that Dr. Riordan had established.[7]

The conference took place in September, attracted 500 people, and was a critical success although it ran a $19,000 deficit after registration fees and button, t-shirt, and bookstore sales of about $13,500.[8] The whole event was orchestrated by about eight staff members, and the personal touch included giving registrants packages of fresh fruit actually hand picked by the organizers. People involved remembered many years later that "no one was overweight at that time." [9] Riordan used his "cough index" as a guide to audience satisfaction, finding that fewer coughs corresponded well with higher speaker ratings. Tracking the number of coughs per time frame compared with the background cough level showed him that the cough index at the conference was low overall.[10] He also noted with pleasure that attendees would come to Wichita, although the nay-sayers had told him that they would not, and that doctors who came to the conference to speak did not depart immediately, but stayed and listened to the other speakers — a pattern that was most uncommon at the standard conference. At most conferences too "the rooms are empty and the conversations were in the hall." Here they attended sessions. Cramer Reed encouraged students at the medical school in Wichita to attend, and there was class credit

---

7 Ibid, Aug. 29, 1977.
8 Ibid, Sept. 19, Nov. 9, 1977.
9 Interview Marilyn Landreth with Craig Miner, Aug. 18, 1999.
10 *Rope*, Oct. 3, 1977.

given to naturopathic students from Oregon who were getting their first two years of education at Kansas Newman. Staff remembered that they were very hungry and ran the suppliers short on food.[11]

The Second International Conference, held in September 1978, was also gratifying to The Center and to the attendees, despite some glitches. A student award competition was added and there were submissions from medical schools all over the country.[12] 200,000 brochures were mailed to health care professionals, nursing schools, medical schools, and dental schools in 11 states. There were three categories in which awards were given: physician-osteopath, nursing schools, and health-related professionals, with a runner-up in each category. In addition there was an overall winner.[13] No names were used of individuals or institutions in the judging, and the efficacy of the evaluation was proved later when many of the winners went on to outstanding scientific achievement. The overall winner received $1,000 and had free attendance at the conference. The money for the awards was given by Sara Welch, who subsequently became a board member at The Center, and was still in that position at the turn of the 21st century at age 90. One night of the conference was always a social occasion at Dr. Riordan's house, where staff and speakers and students interacted casually. One person, Eric Braverman, who won twice, shared with many others the distinction of becoming an MD and doing significant work. Another winner years later had a fire in his house and contacted Dr. Riordan asking if his student award plaque could be replaced, as he valued it so highly. For the year 2000 conference, all the past winners were contacted, and their contributions were impressive. They provided links throughout the country with the standard medical profession.[14]

---

[11] Interview, Dr. Hugh Riordan with Craig Miner, May 27, 1998. Interview Laura Benson, Aug. 18, 1999.
[12] *Rope*, Aug. 12, 1978.
[13] Ibid, April 24, 1978. Interview, Laura Benson and Marilyn Landreth with Craig Miner, Aug. 18, 1999.
[14] Interview, Laura Benson and Marilyn Landreth with Craig Miner, Aug. 18, 1999.

One inconvenience occurred when Jo Ann Pottorff, who had been coordinator of the conference, departed to run Kansas Governor Robert Bennett's reelection campaign for central Kansas.[15] Also disturbing was a death at the conference. Dr. Takahiro Toshii of Tokyo was stricken while presenting an address on his work. Dr Riordan carried him off the stage. Only 50, Toshi had always wanted to come to the United States and because his death occurred while he was presenting on behalf of the medical school for his college, his wife received a pension that was double what she would have received otherwise. Since then, there has been a memorial lecture given at each conference in honor of this man and that striking experience.[16]

Given those conditions, Riordan made it a special point to thank his staff. "As you probably know," he wrote,

> it is my opinion that our staff is made up of exceptionally alert and alive human beings who make the day to day operations of The Center, Laboratory, Institute a really stimulating and worthwhile experience for me. Actually, I know of no other group of people with whom I would rather work. Of course, my opinion is probably biased and therefore open to question. But, after last weekend's Conference there can be no question. Speaker after speaker took the time to come up to me and remark that our staff was the best they had encountered anywhere. Thanks for being you and for working here.

Among the compliments was one from Dr. Denis Burkitt, who was selected by participants as the 2nd annual conference's outstanding speaker. He wrote on his return to England that "I would like to express…my thanks and appreciation for all the efforts you are making to direct proper thoughts to the treatment of man as a whole individual

---

15 *Rope*, Aug. 21, 1978.
16 Letter, Dr. Hugh Riordan to Mrs. Takahiro Yoshii, Sept, 20, 1978 in *Rope*.

and not merely as a chemical machine. You will do more for man than the cardiac by-pass teams will ever accomplish."[17]

Burkitt was indeed the highlight of several conferences with his talk on the seemingly pedestrian topic of "The Importance of High Fiber." What he said, however, was revolutionary and the way that he said it was riveting to the audience. His basic point was that there were many "diseases of civilization" that were costing huge sums in the US and that were virtually unknown in the third world. Burkitt worked in Africa for 43 years without seeing a case of appendicitis. The same was true of gall bladder problems, though gall bladder surgery was the most common abdominal operation in the United States. 1,000 gall bladders were taken out every day of the week in North America, while there was only one operation in five years in Africa. It was a "shattering insult," Burkitt said, that more money is spent taking out gall bladders in the US than the entire medical budget, curative and preventive, on the continent of Africa. What made it particularly insulting was that gall bladder problems could be prevented by the simple expedient of eating a high fiber diet. Burkitt claimed that people "learned" to get coronary heart disease, diabetes, hiatal hernias, varicose veins, hemorrhoids, diverticular disease, and cancers of the bowel by learning to eat an unhealthy diet. None of these need occur.

That was surprising enough, but what really got the attention of listeners was Burkitt's description of the signals of a low-fiber diet and what to do about it in one's personal life. "We are," he would say after showing a few slides with charts of statistics, "a totally constipated nation." He asked how many knew the amount of stool they passed a day, or the average by Americans. Hardly any doctors knew, though Burkitt asked them this unsettling question at conferences regularly. If pressed they guessed about 1.5 pounds. Actually in England and the US the figure was less than 1/4 pound. Americans ate a high fat and low fiber diet, and passed hard stools in relatively small quantities. That was very hard on the intestines, but it was so common that American hotels often installed telephones in bathrooms, knowing that people

---

17 *Rope*, Sept. 25, 1978.

would be spending a lot of time there. Some great things, surely, had been accomplished by constipated people, maybe most famously by Martin Luther, but for most the frustration was not worth it.

Eating fiber, such as contained in whole grains, allowed the body to hold water in the gut, and caused a person to pass large, soft stools that floated. It might be offensive for people to check whether they had "sinkers" or "floaters," but it could have a most significant effect on their future hospital bills. The number of a nation's stools, Burkitt liked to say, was inversely related to the number of its hospitals. He couldn't show people going to the bathroom at a lecture, he said, but the US diet, combined with our type of toilet (people in other parts of the world squatted rather than sitting) meant that we exerted enormous pressure, forcing the stomach up through the diaphragm and causing damage every day. Also with the "ordinary Wichita diet," most of the nutrients were absorbed in the upper part of the intestines, creating a great demand for the production of insulin, an excessive load on the pancreas, and consequently more diabetes.

Salad was not fiber, Burkitt pointed out. Potatoes and parsnips were better. Cattle fodder would be good, but was not generally available in grocery stores. One might try whole wheat bread, high fiber breakfast cereal, and/or a little miller's bran each day. That would "revolutionize bowel behavior." Meat, as another doctor had once said, "should be consumed as a condiment rather than dominating the diet."

None of this was new. Burkitt quoted Dr. T. R. Allison, who, in 1890, had said Americans were constipated because of white bread, and that this caused "headaches" and "miserable feelings." In later times it only got worse as US consumption of sugar and fat rocketed up after 1910. It was time again to look at the causes of things, rather than treat the symptoms. Why clean up the floor constantly from an overflowing sink, Burkitt said, rather than turn off the faucet? Doctors had learned "how to scrub floors and use specialized mops and brushes," but the new medicine had to look for the taps to stop the flood and to break the floor mopper's union.[18]

---

18 Summarized from videotape of Denis Burkitt, "The Importance of High Fiber," presented at Third International Conference on Human Functioning, Sept. 14, 1979, Mabee Library, CIHF.

Burkitt was only one of the speakers at that second conference. A sampling of others suggests the range.

Dr. G. R. Greenwell noted before his audience at Wichita's downtown Century II Convention Center that good health must be earned. Prescriptions should not be for drugs but for lifestyle changes. "Doctors have always thought they had to do something for patients instead of teaching them to do things for themselves. Optimum health is like self-respect — nobody can give it to you, you have to earn it."

Greenwell was from Florida and was the former chair of the AAU sports committee. He had concluded long ago that the American health care system was "bound in irony." It did not teach people to be healthy. For that he blamed money. "People don't mind paying $12,000 for a heart by-pass operation that doesn't change their disease, but they object to spending $200 for a program that can actually alter the cardiovascular disease process." Greenwell had done something about it himself by establishing the Life Clinic, an exercise and fitness center which provided personal assessments and exercise programs, which he thought people, as they became better educated, would demand. Like so many others at the conference, Greenwell appreciated a forum to be heard and the chance to discuss matters with others working in the same area.[19]

Another speaker at the second conference was Dr. Emanual Cheraskin, chair of the Department of Oral Medicine at the University of Alabama Medical Center. Cheraskin became a consultant to The Center. His theme was the abuse of diets — the fad aspect of so-called good health. "If you pine for a figure that's lithe and thin," he told the audience, "and starve through diet after diet to find it, you may end up as mad as a hatter long before you get thin as a rail." Diets ruined marriages, careers, and social life. Even simple changes, if they were wrong, could affect behavior: "one doesn't lose weight, one loses his marbles." Sugar and salt were the great offenders. The typical US citizen ate a teaspoon of sugar every 30-40 minutes around the clock. They got too little vitamin C, vitamin A and calcium. When they missed a meal, as

---

19 *Wichita Eagle Beacon*, Sept. 16, 1978, in History Scrapbook #1, CIHF Archives.

they often did, and their blood sugar dropped, they became sharper-tongued and more irritable — something the world did not need. The American Institute for Family Relations recommended that couples having marital problems have blood sugar tests.

Like the rest of the speakers, Cheraskin was not shy in recommending what could and should be done about it. He called for massive changes in the way American food was grown, marketed and prepared. People should eat more raw or little-cooked food and should "throw out anything that comes in a package." They needed to "vaccinate" themselves with vitamins against the affects of a stripped diet and a hazardous environment. Vitamin C, for example, attacked lead which Americans breathed in the streets every day. The bad news was that it was a serious problem; the good news was that any individual could do something about it with a little knowledge and a little discipline. Cheraskin's book *Psychodietetics* went into The Center's library. [20]

Delores Krieger, a full professor in nursing at New York University, was on that second conference program to discuss therapeutic touch. She had been laughed at for recruiting "Krieger's Krazies" from among nurses, but 4,000 of them had taken her "New Horizons in Medicine" course and thought its precepts fitted their clinical experience. She thought that therapeutic touch was medically sound and should be used in hospitals regularly. "It is an excellent treatment for pain and it accelerates healing.…We're on the edge of a new age where we're beginning to realize that, literally, there is more to a human being than meets the eye. 'Mind,' we're beginning to realize, plays a profound part in life." Touch was no substitute for regular medical care, nor was it "a mystic interaction with a patient, but simply another nursing skill." In meditative healing there occurred "a quiet transfer of energy from healer to patient." Although it looked "absurdly simple," it helped the patient to heal herself. The only failures were among those patients hostile to the process and to the healer.[21]

Dr. Riordan outlined a "five-year plan" in his *Rope* letter in January

---

20 *Wichita Eagle*, Sept. 14, 1978, ibid.
21 *Wichita Eagle Beacon*, Sept. 17, 1978, ibid.

1978. At least it was as close to a plan as a man could devise who did not want any plan to interfere with what he and his colleagues might learn and discover. "Up to this point," he wrote,

> The Center seems to have evolved as the result of particular energy forces (largely in the form of human beings) finding each other almost spontaneously in a way that certainly was not envisioned even short months before the occurrence of each synergism in our growth and development. Thus far, our method of operation, which could be considered loose, is in reality an openness to a variety of input from many, many sources. This is the antithesis of a bureaucracy. It is my hope that our long range planning will not increase our tendency to be bureaucratic and will not in any way diminish our capacity to be open and receptive to the input of energies not envisioned at this point in time. For, in my opinion, what makes The Center a unique entity is our capacity for independence of thought and action in a world in which conformity is so dominating and oppressive in relation to the process. Any long range plans should include an understanding of Doctor Riordan's expected personal odyssey.

Riordan was proud that The Center's agenda was not set by any corporate interest, and that its main supporter, Mrs. Garvey, was sympathetic with so many of his ideas.

Consequently, Riordan proposed to work 77-80 hours a week at The Center when in town, to train executive directors for both The Center and for the Biomedical Synergistics Institute, which was the educational branch. He himself would become the director of the Healthy People Division of The Center, and as such would be much involved in the Personal Health Control program, designed to create a significant database of the characteristics of healthy people and the effects of lifestyle changes upon them. In seven years he planned to become worldwide spokesman for The Center, and in eight years president of the American Holistic Medical Association. The Center itself must expand its staff. It needed a biochemist. It needed to develop more of a volunteer staff. It needed more office space. It needed a new facility, perhaps including growth chambers for hydroponic plants and indoor recreation and housing. There was also an ambitious research agenda including a study of sugar intake, a study of the uses of high dose sodium ascorbate in the elimination of drug withdrawal symptoms, a study to determine the factors involved in the causes of human astigmatism, a study of the correspondence of lung cancer to tobacco use, a study of the correlation between high white count cytotoxicity and leukemia, a study to develop "heavy vegetables" with nutritional content altered by hydroponic feeding of trace elements, the development of a truly normal lab criteria based on those who are actually healthy now instead of on the "crazy idea" that 95% of the population is healthy, and a study to determine the effects of electromagnetic fields on learning and behavior. In education, The Center proposed to develop videotape programs on food preparation, on acupuncture for the relief of pain, on hyperactivity and food coloring, and on finger temperature and biofeedback. It would publish a public newsletter and possibly a scientific journal.[22]

The connections made with the standard medical profession were modest and tenuous. And in the case of insurance reimbursement, which The Center in its original plan was depending upon, the expected result did not occur.

Some rumblings on the insurance front appeared late in 1976. The Center got the news that Dr. Earl Vivino, an MD/PhD cardiologist, had been expelled from the Washington, DC Medical Society for allegedly ordering unnecessary medical tests, a favorite bugbear of the insurance industry.

There was a possible similarity to The Center. "We are certainly at the forefront of doing tests which would not fall under 'accepted standards,' and many of our psychiatric colleagues would view our testing

---

22 *Rope*, Jan., 1978.

as unnecessary in light of their level of awareness. Most other physicians would concur since very few even consider nutrition in their work."

It was difficult to achieve a clear understanding with Blue Cross/Blue Shield, which administered Medicare, that The Center was providing a good cost-benefit ratio by curing people. The Center's complete evaluation cost less than 10 hours of psychotherapy or four days of typical psychiatric hospitalization.[23] One alternative would be to limit the number of Medicare patients. Another was to protest. Riordan wrote a letter in November 1976 to the executive Vice President of the American Medical Association. He pointed out that recent AMA testimony before Congress stated that "it is impossible to substitute for the individual physician's judgment when dealing with an individual patient in an individual setting with an individual set of conditions." That was heartening to Riordan — "it gave me the reassurance that it is perhaps not necessary to practice medicine by committee." [24]

In December, Riordan had considerable contact with a Blue Cross representative. He described The Center's lab capabilities. The Center lab was using Pfeiffer's Brain Bio Center in New Jersey as a model, and had sophisticated means for testing trace minerals, kryptopyrrole, and polyamines. It had added cytotoxic testing for food sensitivities of the type pioneered in St. Louis and also a computerized system of analyzing plasma and urine for 46 amino acids. The Center had developed several innovative techniques itself, including a way of determining the clinical significance of hypoglycemia in any individual by correlating blood sugar levels with plasma and urinary ascorbic acid levels. The lab was certified by state and federal agencies. One area hospital and two mental health centers were using the Bio Center lab. Its fees were less expensive than most because it was partially underwritten, but its practice of quoting package prices for interrelated tests, as well as doing tests that were unusual, led inevitably to fractures with the insurance carriers over what was "necessary." Riordan emphasized that Center physician fees were fixed and did not fluctuate with their uti-

---

23 Ibid, n.d. [c. Dec. 1, 1976].
24 Letter, Riordan to James Sammons, Nov. 28, 1976, in *Rope*.

lization of the lab. Therefore they had no financial conflict of interest in ordering tests.

What kind of diagnosis was used? That was "a difficult area." A recent patient was hospitalized for depression, and The Center found she had food sensitivities and related hypoglycemia, both of which it had been able to correct, relieving the depression. But there was a catch. "Unfortunately at the present time there is no acceptable diagnosis to properly reflect her impairment. Therefore, although she is not a 'psychiatric case,' but rather a 'biochemical case,' she is considered a psychiatric case by Blue Shield-Blue Cross and consequently has been denied benefits." At that time The Center had three people under treatment, including a physician's son, "who were clearly mentally disturbed — except they weren't." All were treated for low levels of vitamin C and low utilization. The insurance carrier, however, thought The Center should not even do a vitamin C test since it was not a recognized test for schizophrenia. "And, appallingly, there was little concern that the patient was free from hallucination, functioning better than in years, and not in need of psychotherapy or tranquilizing drugs."[25]

There were frequent examples of this type, and The Center was constantly trying to explain them to hospitals as well as insurance companies. There was chart #B576317 at St. Francis in April 1979, for example. This patient had symptoms of depression, mental confusion, and weakness. She was too confused to maintain on an open floor, and the internal medicine consultant said her problem was "hysterical neurosis." Her hometown physician had indicated adrenal insufficiency, which tests did not reveal. However, The Center lab discovered her plasma C level was zero and her serum copper to zinc ratio was 155/85. Normally copper to zinc should be one to one. When these two biochemical deviations from normal were treated, she was fine. "The question I would like to ask," Riordan wrote the St. Francis Psychiatric Department Committee, "is what diagnosis or diagnoses do you feel would be acceptable in this case — depressive neurosis? — adult scurvy — copper zinc imbalance?"[26]

---

25 Letter, Riordan to Graham Bailey, Dec. 6, 1976, in *Rope*.
26 Letter, Riordan to J. Luis Ibarra April 16, 1979 in *Rope*.

By the summer of 1977, a few tests were being paid for by insurance.[27] In November 1977, Riordan appeared for four hours before 100 people representing the Kansas SRS in 19 counties. The president of that organization had received calls questioning the appropriateness of paying a "quack like Doctor Riordan with state funds." The callers were told that no state funds were involved, that the SRS did not think Riordan was a quack, and that he would talk to whomever wanted to listen. His talk was taped by cable TV in Abilene where it was given.[28]

The talk went well. However, the more The Center grew, and the more publicity it got, the more violent were some of the attacks on it. Late in 1977 an "incredible" letter came from a psychiatrist. Riordan thought that "the preposterous high handedness of the demands" was evidence that The Center was shaking up things. However, it was disturbing too.[29]

And it was not totally isolated. In 1979, Riordan confided in Mrs. Garvey about a particular incident. A woman volunteering in the Personal Health Control program was the wife of an officer of the Sedgwick County Medical Society. One day, the woman appeared in Dr. Riordan's office, burst into tears, and said she could no longer work at The Center because her husband disapproved. Her husband, at least in Riordan's translation, thought it was inappropriate for the wife of a prominent physician "to be urging people to stay healthy when doctors made their money from sick people." Second, her husband was fearful of losing referrals in reprisal for her support of The Center's Personal Health Control program.

Riordan was not unsympathetic. He had been threatened with loss of income himself several times. Once was when his own wife's involvement in the La Leche League, which promoted breast feeding, led some doctors to tell Riordan they would no longer make referrals to him. Riordan being Riordan, he told those "delightful doctors to go ____

---

27 Ibid, Oct. 7, 1977.
28 Ibid, Nov. 8, 1977.
29 Ibid, Dec. 12, 1977.

themselves. Then I joined La Leche as a member of their international professional advisory board where I have served for some 18 years." [30]

Dr. Riordan remained disgusted about these events twenty years later. Insurance paid for procedures, he concluded with sadness, not for results. "There is no insurance form that ever asks, 'How did you do?' which is tragic."[31] Riordan remembered: "We were lied to regularly, and our patients were lied to." He felt there was outright specific prejudice. Insurance would not reimburse The Center for amino acid profiles, for example, but when Riordan and Hinshaw sent their own samples to an insurance-approved lab in California for no reason at all, the bill was immediately paid by Blue Cross/Blue Shield. [32]

Despite these setbacks, Riordan continued to try to convince the insurance carriers. In June 1978, he wrote to the Blue Cross board that one piece of evidence that The Center was not doing unnecessary tests was the high ratio of abnormal findings to normal results in those tests. The ratio of abnormal results was much higher than in those labs that were paid by insurance without question. "I cannot imagine," Riordan wrote to the insurance people, "how there can be any question as to the appropriateness of test selection at the Bio Center Laboratory based upon these statistics."

Of course there was. Riordan argued that The Center operated on a medical model and "shied away from anecdotal reports." Its $500 package arrangement for a two-day stay was only for out-of-state patients. It reduced the need for later appointments and travel. Eleven distinguished physicians familiar with The Center were willing to testify before the insurance officers "or in court as the need may arise." [33]

There was no relief. In the fall of 1978, The Center was working on a way of establishing "medical necessity" for its tests as defined by the health insurance industry. The chair of the Blue Cross/Blue Shield physician utilization board explained that "medical necessity concepts

---

30 Letter, Riordan to Olive W. Garvey, April 2, 1979, Office Files, CIHF Archives.
31 Interview, Dr. Hugh Riordan with Craig Miner, June 10, 1998.
32 Interview, Dr. Hugh Riordan with Craig Miner, May 27, October 22, 1998.
33 Letter, Riordan to Henry Meiners, June 5, 1978 in *Rope*.

are based upon an assumption that laboratory services ordered on a patient are based upon some kind of appropriate diagnosis or at least a significant preliminary diagnosis. Batteries of tests and screening tests that have no specific relation to the patient's symptomology and preliminary diagnoses are not considered medically necessary." That definition was of course a problem for holistic medicine which might look for causes of a disease in non-traditional places, and it was a problem for preventative testing and treatment, so much a part of alternative medicine.[34]

Riordan wrote an extensive response to that. Maybe the visitors to The Center for the insurance company had "provided you with the impression that we are performing extensive biochemical screening of normal individuals who just happen to drop by." That was not the case. "Should you choose to become familiar with our work," Riordan wrote, the head of the physician utilization board would find that The Center did not provide primary care. The ticket there was past medical treatment with an unsatisfactory outcome — that is, the "medically necessary" tests did not work, and the "proper" diagnosis did not relate to the underlying cause for that kind of patient. The Center collected an extensive medical history, including multiple evaluations, before it ordered any lab work. It was not unusual to have 2-4 inches of medical records to review. It did not repeat what had been done. The high percentage of abnormal results showed there was a relation between the tests and the suspected pathology. If it had a high percentage of normals as in the case of skull x-rays, chest x-rays and upper G.I. series, the insurers would "swoop down" on it about too many tests. Riordan wanted to have face-to-face discussions on the matter. The insurers did not. He wanted to appear at a board meeting with his supporting physicians; they did not want him to. "This leaves a very high degree of frustration," he wrote, "and very few options."[35]

After 1979, the insurance question, which had occupied a good deal of The Center's archives, almost disappeared as a topic of discus-

---

34 Letter, Dr. Glenn Bair to Riordan, Sept. 6, 1978, *Rope*.
35 Letter, Riordan to Glenn Bair, Oct. 11, 1978, in *Rope*.

sion. The class action suit was never filed, as Riordan did not believe it would be a good use of energy even if the outcome were positive, and other matters took up all the time and energy the staff had to give. There was a proud little note in 1984 that for the first time that year an insurance company had referred a client to The Center for evaluation and treatment — in this instance for back pain.[36] And there was a more extensive wail in 1987, when it was noted that an insurance company had paid thousands for outpatient and hospital care for two years for a young lady without improvement. It then refused to pay The Center's modest fee even though the patient dramatically improved and returned to full function. Her father was so incensed that he threatened to sue. That generated more inquiry from the company, to which Riordan responded. He sent a series of articles dealing with the biochemistry of depression in people like this patient, and commented that

> from my perspective as a clinician who sees only people who have been treated medically elsewhere without success, I find your request for information supporting what we do to be most frustrating, albeit standard. What you should be interested in when deciding whether to pay a bill for one of your insured is how they do — what kind of result are they having. Instead you pay for process however dismal the outcome may be. As the result, you pay enormous amounts for established but ineffective processes because they are the accepted thing to do instead of paying for what works as in this case. As a consequence, countless people suffer because physicians, in part coerced by reimbursable insurance payments, find it easier to 'do things right' than doing the right thing.[37]

The Center did make a serious attempt in 1989 before the state

---

36 Ibid, Dec. 3, 1984.
37 Ibid, April 20, 1987.

insurance commissioner to reopen the question of remuneration. Otherwise, excepting the occasional outburst, there was silence, and new determination.

Insurance was perhaps the key factor in The Center's moving away from a mission involving serious interaction with the standard medical profession and toward a more ambitious dream of independent, no-compromise existence until such time as the profession moved its way. Riordan was able to write in 1984 that The Center had grown "without a single dime of government tax money and its attendant bureaucratic intervention and control, without even a single strand of string attached to or from any special interest group." It was a bitter pill at first to swallow as The Center struggled for funding and hesitated to ask Mrs. Garvey for more, but in hindsight, it seemed to the staff that such independence was, like so many things, destined to be.[38]

The huge agenda outlined in the 1978 "five year plan" was the result of an ever firmer philosophy, which Riordan had embellished partly as the result of conversation with innovative physicians all over the world who were contacted by the new educational branch of The Center. The new medicine needed to alter significantly "our degree of wellness and our capacity for longevity past middle age. We know that a positive change is overdue. Developing the capacity to effect such a change and the capacity to effect a positive change in the level of health and vitality for all ages would seem to be a worthy project for The Center to undertake." To do so required more focus on preventative medicine. "This is the process of developing an understanding that survival and the quality of survival are directly related to how closely we are able to approximate internally what is optimal biochemically. Predictive medicine, which may be defined as the clinical discipline designed to anticipate disease in man, emphasizes primary prevention (prevention of occurrence). It should be possible for us to begin to effect positive changes in vitality and longevity and to collect hard data by doing a pilot study of at least 100 people." [39]

---

38 Ibid, Dec. 24, 1984.
39 Ibid, Jan., 1978.

That study, which Garvey funded with a special appropriation of $300,000, was called Personal Health Control, and was the first real public program of The Center. The original idea was to study 1,000 people, to collect full information on their "normal" biochemistry, and then to introduce lifestyle changes and note the results. It was supposed to be a national program, drawing 100 people from each of ten Health, Education, and Welfare Districts, and measuring their improved health in the future by tracking changes in sick leave days.[40]

Riordan was interested in sick leave and its abuses. In 1978 he eliminated sick leave for employees of The Center, and used funds formerly spent on flowers for those in the hospital for sending flowers to the desks of those who were working. He then instituted a program of positive reinforcement, giving certain planned days off as a reward for being well and staying on the job. The Center did not have a retirement plan either because, Riordan wrote, "it is antithetical to enhanced human functioning to require people to stop working when they may be most capable."[41]

In Riordan's mind the main reason for eliminating sick leave was that it encouraged lying and poor health. Most people had a conscience, so if they called in sick they thought they ought to feel at least a little sick, and that caused more illness than necessary. The staff had many questions, such as "do you expect me to crawl to work?" The answer was no, but if one had a headache it was just as well to have it amid supportive people. If it were a viral infection, the person was contagious 10-14 days earlier, and at The Center could get vitamin C to cure it quickly. During the first six months of the program sick days off were reduced by 75%. Subsequently The Center instituted "health incentives" in which people were paid extra for accomplishing certain health related behaviors, such as drinking enough water, walking, retaining the ideal weight, and annually writing a positive statement

---

40 Interview, Dr. Hugh Riordan with Craig Miner, June 3, 1998. Hugh Riordan, "'In Search of Wellness:' A New Look at Yourself," *Wichita BMC News & Views* (June, 1979), vol. 2, #2, in History Scrapbook #1, CIHF Archives.
41 *Rope*, Aug. 12, 1978.

about every co-worker they knew. Looking at good things about other people tended to make the staff feel better about themselves. And trying healthy practices on themselves not only made that habitual, but made the staff more aware of the needs of patients and The Center's method of dealing with them. Staff would sometimes read and review books, the more sophisticated presentations getting the larger incentive bonuses. Blue Cross later said that The Center staff at the end of the century had one of the lowest rates of utilization of services of any organization its size, despite being older than the average group. For the year 2000, it was given a 7% reduction in health premium cost, while most organizations in its category had their rates raised by 8%.[42] Personal Health Control was the next step and was to be marketed to companies partly as a means of keeping employees productive and at work rather than on sick leave.

In June 1978 Dr. Everett DeWhitt, a 44-year-old PhD from the University of Oklahoma in Health Physics, Civil Engineering and Environmental Sciences, was employed as associate director of the PHC project. Riordan described his working conditions to him as "probably poor for two years and with too little space, too little staff and too much to do." Responsibilities: "Although your titles suggest your primary areas of responsibility, you will be expected to assist with your expertise, brain power, perception or physical energy when considered necessary by the Director."[43]

Personal Health Control did not work just as planned. It was to be a two stage process. An initial group was to be fewer than 10 healthy people. These had to be within 10% of ideal weight, not have smoked for three years, consume no more than 3 oz. of alcohol a week, have an exercise program and sleep well. The idea was to get optimum lab values for really healthy people as contrasted with "normal" people as 95% of the population was usually defined. Then, in stage 2, a group of 1,000 people nationwide representative of the general population

---

[42] Interview, Dr. Hugh Riordan with Craig Miner, October 22, 1998. Interview, Laura Benson and Marilyn Landreth with Craig Miner, Aug. 18, 1999.
[43] *Rope*, June 11, 12, 1978.

PYRAMID ON THE PRAIRIE

was to do a health-improving regimen at home to show how much healthier even these could be.[44]

The changes came in the second stage. When it was announced in the *Wichita Eagle* that The Center was looking for volunteers who would be asked to participate in a program to enhance their degree of wellness, nearly 800 Wichitans signed up in a matter of days, and there were bitter complaints from those who had to be turned away. As a result, most of those involved in Personal Health Control were chosen from Kansas, with only about 75 from the rest of the country. A second part of the plan was that all the participants would be working people, so that the results of the program could be evaluated in changes in sick leave time. However, again the demand was great from those who were homemakers, and therefore some participants, as it turned out, were not in paid positions. However, the process and the goal remained the same.

That process was to study the PHC people for fourteen weeks (the actual project turned out to be twelve), changing one thing about their lifestyle in each of those weeks. They received a kit with instructions and forms for feedback. It was not so much a matter of asking people to change their behavior as allowing them to do so. When they were given a pedometer and asked to report on their walking, they tended to walk further. And attitudes changed also. At the exit interview when asked what was their most significant health help, medication dropped from the #1 position it had held at the beginning to #5. It was clearly an educational as well as a research project.[45]

The packets contained something of everything people at The Center had learned. There were exercises with high-fiber diet, containing not only instructions as to what to do, but explanations on why, taken largely from the studies of Dr. Denis Burkitt on the "diseases of civilization." While using three tablespoons of extra wheat bran a day, the PHC participant could read that "it is possible to laboriously scrutinize the minutest weaknesses in the defense system and yet overlook a glaring and unnoticed defect." Those who focused "arc-lights on protein,

---

44 *Rope*, n.d. [Spring, 1979]
45 Interview, Dr. Hugh Riordan with Craig Miner, June 3, 1998.

vitamin and calorie needs, and on the disadvantageous changes in the quality of our fats and cooking oils, for the most part considered fiber as an inert, valueless and disposable component of foods and consequently tended to disregard it as a virtual contaminant." It was anything but. Among the diseases that were linked to low fiber in the standard American diet were coronary heart disease, diverticular disease of the colon, appendicitis, colon-rectal cancer, diabetes and obesity. Eliminating these through diet would bring huge financial savings as well as the relief of enormous suffering.[46]

Would people question the advice? Certainly. Was there a huge database of tests confirming the efficacy of all of it? No. Should people then wait to try some of these common-sense solutions? The answer to that varied, but to the PHC participants The Center quoted Mark 44:27: "A man scatters seed on the land….the seed sprouts and grows…how, he does not know." We are, the material in PHC packet #2 pointed out, always acting on "reasonable association." Had the seed planter of old inhibited his action "until the intricacies of seed germination were intellectually grasped, he and his family would soon have starved." Maybe you won't like to "sneak a peak" at your bowel movements just before flushing, nor think at first it matters whether they sink or float, but has anything else so simple been suggested with such a prospect of improving your health?[47]

Personal Health Control made many friends for The Center and continued for several years. One man, who weighed 300 pounds, wrote that his family was a little tired of his talking about fiber and remembering to take his vitamin C, but that he felt great. He had not played tennis in years, but that week played 20 games with his son.[48] Another man wrote that he was substituting fruits for refined sugars, and changing from sweet breakfast rolls to whole wheat toast. "Bananas at $.30 a pound are considerably more economical than steak at $2.50 a pound."[49]

---

46 PHC packet #2 in *Rope,* n.d. [Feb., 1979].
47 Personal Health Control, Packet #2 [Feb., 1979] in *Rope*.
48 Ibid, May 7, 1979.
49 Ibid, Dec. 18, 1979.

In the second year of PHC, The Center collected comments from the participants on their motivation and what they expected to gain. The answers provided a cross-section of the attractions of The Center's style of medicine generally, and a survey of why the new medicine was gaining nationally. "Everything that ails me is stress connected," wrote a housemother, 62 years old. "A relaxed body and mind, a feeling of well-being and elimination of the feeling 'I don't know what's wrong with me, but I feel terrible,'" was the response of a 37-year-old secretary. A technical writer wrote: "Good health means peace of mind." A teacher said: "I am curious about how change in diet will affect the way I feel and act." A housewife thought the best thing would be "presence of mind through better health knowledge." A secretary hoped to "get into the 'health habit' as I've done other habits." To a 28-year-old teacher, the goal was simply put: "Control!" [50]

The Personal Health Control program was thus the beginning of the "co-learner" practice with patients. Riordan had noticed that "most people are not aware that they are responsible for things," and did not want his patients to be that way. He wanted them to respect the knowledge of the physician, but not be intimidated by it, and he wanted them to understand their ailments and to read widely on them. In the early years most of the contributions to The Center were anonymous. These came from people who believed in what it was doing, but were afraid to be associated with it publicly. That changed as the education program and the involvement of people through programs like Personal Health Control got The Center out of the realm of myth. It attracted what Riordan called a "pretty sharp" clientele. He never liked to see people who were brought to The Center by a well-meaning friend, but who did not themselves understand why they were there.[51] Any patient who complained was refunded his or her money, and The Center prided itself on having no lawsuits filed against it in its first four years.[52] Riordan also was aware early that the quality of care required

---

50 Patient comments in *Rope*, n.d. [Jan., 1979].
51 Interview, Dr. Hugh Riordan with Craig Miner, June 10, 1998.
52 *Rope*, Feb. 5, 1979, Jan. 18, 1980.

meant that there had to be a limited number of patients, no matter how much "mass production" would contribute to the bottom line. It had to be small enough that the question on the initial survey about what patients would like to be called meant that they were actually called that by the whole staff. This smallness was insured partly because The Center could only handle so many and refused to add doctors just to expand, and partly because the goal was to dismiss patients by curing them or teaching them to treat themselves. This meant that, while the number of patients currently being seen there was small, the number who had been seen and influenced by this organization became eventually large indeed. When a "patient" became a co-learner it was a "whole different world."[53]

One of those earliest in the PHC program was Carolyn Kortge, then a reporter for the *Wichita Eagle* and later a writer on fitness subjects, including the 1998 book *The Spirited Walker*. Kortge was one of six volunteers recruited in the spring of 1978 for a pilot study for Personal Health Control, and she wrote about it for the newspaper.

She went to The Center, Kortge wrote, having not eaten since midnight, and having had no coffee or cigarettes, to give what seemed like innumerable vials of blood. It was "a grisly endurance exercise that was an unsettling introduction to what lay ahead during a three-month study of nutrition, body chemistry and wellness. For three months, I gave up my arms to endless needles, hurled unwilling muscles across racquetball courts, shunned red meat for two weeks, sugar for two more and went with no food at all for two days. I took extra doses of vitamin C, measured my footsteps with a pedometer and relaxed to a tape-recorded voice. It was all in the name of health and self-discovery, and I discovered even before the pilot program began that self-discovery is often painful....I wondered at the wisdom of my decision to donate my healthy, happy, living body to the rigors of science." She got "cold, dizzy, cranky, and tired" only to find out in the end that "I am hopelessly normal." That was the type Riordan was seeking. He wanted people who were well and he wanted to see what they do to be well, and how they could be more well.

---

53 Interview, Dr. Hugh Riordan with Craig Miner, June 10, 1998.

In Kortge's case "chocolate, coffee and cigarettes showed up as foods my body fights." She gave up two of the three right away. She learned how to listen to her body, and that would be a life-long benefit.[54] "It's a discovery, an odyssey, for the individual, "Riordan told the press. "If one person wants to salt his eggs and another wants to use no salt at all, that's fine. We want the information from them about what's going on." It was not necessary for a person to run 20 miles a day to affect health. Instead "mini-lifestyle changes," like parking farther away from the door, would do if followed consistently. [55]

PHC training was not made into a movie, though Riordan talked about it with a Hollywood producer and sought industrial clients to fund that. There was a half hour documentary made on it for local television. It did create much favorable local publicity for The Center and the philosophy behind it. Dr. Riordan, of course, was a reporter's dream to interview. There was always fear among the staff that the eventual story might be unfriendly and/or distorted. However, the media was a Riordan specialty, both directly and indirectly through his political work in the late 1960s and early 1970s. The risk of distortion was not so great as the risk of failing to get a message out at all. And PHC, with its lure of free health care, provided a wonderful opportunity for community involvement. By the beginning of 1979 there was a waiting list and The Center was trying to get funds from the charity account generated from the refinancing of the Wichita Waterworks bonds. The goal for that application was to provide Personal Health Control for 1% of Wichita's population (that would be 2,630 people), a program The Center thought would make an astounding difference. PHC was, The Center publicity said, "a program which is designed to benefit participants of any age, in any walk of life and at any level of personal wellness." [56]

---

54 Carolyn Kortge, "One Personal Health Odyssey," *Wichita Eagle-Beacon*, Aug. 13, 1978.
55 Hugh Riordan, "'In Search of Wellness: A New Look at Yourself," *Wichita BMC News & Views* (June, 1979), vol 2, #2, in History Scrapbook #1, CIHF Archives.
56 *Rope*, n.d. [Jan., 1979].

The PHC program was encouraging. Many were on the new road, and many wanted, at least, to hear about The Center. It trained its first full-time volunteer in the spring of 1978, and the PHC program and the conferences got considerable publicity for the little complex of offices on Douglas and on Oliver.[57] But when people went to The Center, it was not exactly a "center" — not even close, physically. Its staff was all over the place, communication was imperfect, and the public atmosphere suggested a small standard operation that was struggling to survive.

Sometime in 1977, Dr Riordan had a dream — not a waking thought, but an actual dream. In it he saw a Center on a large rural acreage and with innovative architecture, including domes and a pyramid. Upon awakening he took some notes. Being stimulated to think architecturally by that dream, he started observing closely in his travels where and how institutions were housed. He was impressed by Buckminster Fuller's geodesic dome structures, and the claims for them in strength and energy efficiency. Building such structures would not only be practical, but would reflect The Center's innovative philosophy on health in its physical home. Riordan, too, always imagined a series of low, "human-sized" buildings rather than one large, imposing, "government" type structure. Government buildings were designed to represent authority and to enforce respect. The Center should be designed to facilitate the new type of interaction that it imagined the future would bring between patients and physicians. It should reflect the findings of science and it should incorporate the warmness of its humane mission. Riordan saw a neurosurgeon's 45 foot dome in El Centro, California, that he liked, and he was impressed that it had survived a major earthquake. Tests of geodesic domes at Wichita State University's wind tunnel demonstrated that a 1/4 mile wide tornado would just lift over it without damage. He hired a consultant who recorded 43 hours of audio tapes on different architectural concepts for what Riordan began to call "The Master Facility." Skylights became a feature early. We must, Riordan thought, always be "connected to the universe and have some sense of where we

---

57 *Rope*, March 13, 1978.

are." And he loved the fact that the domes would not be boxes. There are no rectangles in nature.[58]

In November 1977 a group of Kansas State University architecture students worked on ideas for building a physical home for The Center on 90 acres of alfalfa field that Mrs. Garvey owned on North Hillside street, beyond Wichita State University. KSU landscape architecture students had won many awards in recent years, and Riordan wanted to use their ideas along with those of the local planning firm of Oblinger-Smith corporation to develop the very best look and function. Susan Gray was the student who actually made the winning drawings for the site.[59]

For a long time, the dream remained a dream. But, slowly, as circumstances drove The Center into its own corner and the Garvey support strengthened, it became plausible and finally real. Patient fees in 1977 had been over $155,000; that was encouraging.[60]

And the discouragements, while regular, could be overcome. In 1979, struggling with some colleague criticism, Riordan got a letter from a supportive colleague including a quotation from Lao Tzu:

> How can a man's life keep its course
> If he will not let it flow?
> Those who flow as life flows know
> They need no other force:
> They feel no wear, they feel no tear
> They need no mending, no repair.

Maybe that was it. Riordan wrote to Mrs. Garvey on that occasion that he liked to think "that my constitution is such that, whatever the pressure, I would not succumb to the belief system that seems to be operative in Doctor _____'s life . Yet, the pressures for not deviating from what is financially most rewarding — to be one of the boys even though you know the boys are wrong — seems to be

---

58 Interview, Dr. Hugh Riordan with Craig Miner, May 27, 1998.
59 *Rope*, Nov. 21, 1977.
60 Ibid, March 6, 1978.

ever present in society."⁶¹ Her support made the difference for him. She wrote him back: "It is, indeed, a complicated world, whatever the category." She had every expectation "that what it [The Center] accomplishes will have more impact on the future than any other money I have ever spent."⁶²

Riordan met with the extended Garvey family in March 1978, in Arizona. He found them and their advisor Bob Page and his wife "vigorous, intelligent people who possess a high degree of spirit and individualism."⁶³ In April, Warren Oblinger, Riordan, and a KSU student, met to go over plans. If what they discussed could be done, Riordan thought, The Center could be a national attraction for its look alone. "There is a possibility that the electric ground and sky-train units can be powered by windmill energy." There were unique low cost tunnels to connect the domes and "exciting" landscaping concepts.⁶⁴ Naturally, not all of that plan was ever implemented, but it was a firm direction and a goal to which a price tag could be attached.

That dream and that price tag led to another significant change. Beginning in 1980, The Center for the Improvement of Human Functioning became known as the Olive W. Garvey Center for the Improvement of Human Functioning. It was a mouthful, but to those involved it seemed it had to be. The Center had by then seen over 3,000 patients and had 2,500 active files.⁶⁵ "Our track record," Riordan wrote Garvey, "has spanned a sufficient period of time that I believe we should start telling the world that we are here."⁶⁶

The Center had an income, but not nearly enough to replace its crowded facilities or to try seriously to live up to its vision. Mrs. Garvey never promised that she could support any dream or that she could or would support The Center forever. But she was willing to carry it through to the next step of building something in

---

61 Letter, Riordan to Olive W. Garvey, April 2, 1979, Office Files, CIHF Archives.
62 Letter, Olive W. Garvey to Riordan, April 6, 1979, ibid.
63 *Rope*, March 6, 1978.
64 Ibid, April 17, 1978.
65 Ibid, Jan. 28, 1980.
66 Letter, Riordan to Olive W. Garvey, June 8, 1979, Office Files, CIHF Archives.

her alfalfa field that would get the attention of Wichita, and maybe someday the world. It would attract at first by the way it looked, but all hoped eventually by what it was. Dr. Riordan and Mrs. Garvey had an understanding from the first, and in the early 1980s it was to reach its zenith of possibility.

"It now is clear," Riordan wrote Garvey, "to many who had other hopes that we are not likely to fade away. We have moved from a position of an easily ignored entity to a position of being heard and being listened to by an ever increasing number of people. We are no longer the fly on the horse's rump which, though pesky, is easily removed by the switch of a tail. We are, instead, becoming a formidable force which will have to be accepted or reckoned with." He was embarrassed always to ask Garvey for money, but it was easier now "because we are doing a good job." The Center and its people were on the verge of becoming "a great international center."

Chapter Four
One of a Kind

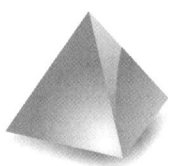

With a campus in its future, and with more substantial funding coming from Mrs. Garvey on that and other fronts, The Center moved to a considerably higher and lonelier profile. Early in 1980, for example, it took on the food editor at the *Wichita Eagle*, concerning her comments in a February 11 article entitled "Is White Bread Bad for You?" White bread, which lent itself marvelously to mechanization, had been around for a century, and the consuming public so much adapted to its soft crust, its texture "with the resiliency of a rubber sponge," its bleached color and its uniform, toaster fitted, pre-sliced size, that generations had regarded it as a thoroughly modern food. Sylvester Graham's protests in the 1830s that the new bread had negative effects on health, down to eliminating productive chewing, fell mostly on deaf ears, and he was remembered in the 20th century as the "inventor" of a graham cracker, which by then had been corrupted into a sweet snack.[1] The *Eagle* article implied that the only ingredient lacking in white compared with whole grain bread was fiber. The writer

---

1 For an entertaining summary of the development of white bread in US industry see Siegfried Giedion, *Mechanization Takes Command* (New York: WW Norton & Company, 1969), pp. 179-208. First published in 1948.

said that "one should disregard those who say that it is not nutritious." The standard loaf had been enriched and fortified and cost only about 1/4 as much as whole grain bread. Yes, in the 1980s there was a health food fad and whole grains were "fashionable." They seemed natural, but how much value did they have really?

The CIHF responded that "unfortunately for the literate public untrue statements such as that one about the quality of white and whole grain flours appear in the printed word with great regularity." If the food editor's source was the US Department of Agriculture's booklet *Nutritive Value of Foods,* it was understandable that she might have been misled. That publication showed nutritive values of white and whole wheat bread that were not very different except for calcium, phosphorous and potassium. The equivalency, however, was only because nutrients lost during refining were replaced with manufactured supplements. Looking at the *Nutrition Almanac,* one could find a vast difference in micronutrients such as zinc, selenium, magnesium, and biotin. These were important to everyone, but particularly to teens with acne or mid-life men with enlarging prostates. And of course anyone who thought that "only fiber" was not of any importance had not been listening to Dr. Burkitt.[2] Several of The Center's staff met personally with the newspaper's food editor, and there was a 90-minute exchange of views. She was given a copy of Williams's *Wonderful World,* and she was added to The Center's mailing list.[3] In Wichita, the public discussion of the topic of nutrition was never thereafter to be the same.

Other media were of interest also. A program like that of The Center depended heavily on education and individual responsibility, and many of the impressions the public had about health were coming through the print and electronic media. In 1980 The Center sponsored a TV program "The Feminine Mistake" about the dangers of smoking.[4] But the great breakthrough in TV was the production by The Center

---

2 *Rope*, Feb. 18, 1980.
3 Ibid, Feb. 25, 1980.
4 Ibid, March 10, 1980.

of an original program called "One of a Kind." It had its origin in the groundswell of interest by youngsters in the PHC program, which was designed for adults. The TV program thus became a kind of Personal Health Control for children.[5]

Obviously, the fact that Dr. Riordan had been in the audio-visual business for several years had much to do with the video documentation of the international conferences and with the fact that a medical center would find itself in any position even to propose producing its own television program. Preparation, however, requires opportunity, and opportunity came, as it did so often, from a person helped by the medical end of The Center's work. Carolyn Kortge was a Personal Health Control participant, and it helped The Center's cause a great deal that she was also a writer for the *Wichita Eagle*. Also among PHC participants was the president of KARD TV, Channel 3 in Wichita, Frank Chappel. The result of their experience at The Center and of Riordan's talking to these two was that in 1980 channel 3 offered The Center free studio time to produce its own children's program on health after having given it free documentary coverage on Personal Health Control. There was a catch: the time was from 12-3 a.m. But with the unusual employee relations situation and the high motivation at The Center, that did not present an impossible obstacle. There was also a financial barrier. When Riordan announced that his budget for 13 episodes of "One of a Kind," was $130,000 for a program which was to include original music, costumed characters and elaborate sets, and which was to compete on *commercial*, not educational television, experienced people in the field and several foundations that might have otherwise supported it laughed out loud. That was about the usual cost of a simple 30-minute interview program. But, as The Center's mantra went, "While others were saying 'It cannot be done,' it was done." The money, as usual, came from Olive Garvey, because perceptually she understood the best way to improve the health of the country was to get the children involved.[6]

---

5 Interview, Marilyn Landreth and Laura Benson with Craig Miner, Aug. 18, 1999.
6 Interview, Dr. Hugh Riordan with Craig Miner, June 3, 1998.

The agreement for "One of a Kind" was signed in May 1980. Some presence on Channel 3 started soon, with segments of "For the Health of it with Doctor Hugh" running weekly for 90 seconds on the noon news beginning in the summer of 1980.[7] In August, Myrliss Hershey, PhD, who was a professor at WSU, joined The Center as associate director of both Health Related Programs and the Biomedical Synergistics Institute.[8] Hershey worked 18-hr. days, was to have much to do with the TV program, and doubtless was much better known among the young residents of Wichita for her role as the Wise Woman in the Cave on "One of a Kind" than for any of her academic achievements.[9] She did it partly for Riordan, whom she described as "an entrepreneur, but with humanitarian reasons."[10] By the time of the 4th International Conference in September, the episodes were near completion.[11] Ads appeared the next month, telling the target audience of 5 to 12-year-olds about a cast of characters which included the host Rainbow Lady; Barbara the Zoo Lady; U2Me2; Tracy the Tree; the Wise Old Owl; the Space Doctor (NASA physician Dr. Charles Berry, a Center consultant); the Nutrition Magician; Moore the Troubadour; Karla the Clown (played by eventual Broadway musical star Karla Burns); Mary Myba, the exercise coach (Move Your Body Around); and Cool Cat. ONEderland with its wondrous Enchanted Tree was the scene, and there were 30 songs. The first half-hour show aired on KARD and its translator affiliates around Kansas on October 18.[12]

The show itself was clean, darling and useful — yet people watched it. There was Dr. Hugh on news center 1 answering questions about health. He was a cloth puppet that looked exactly like Riordan, and of course, the real man did the voice over. The newsman who interviewed him was a dog. The Gatekeeper to Rainbow ONEderland talked with various other velour puppets. In one episode a Kangaroo and a Dragon

---

7 *Rope*, July 21, 1980.
8 Ibid, Aug. 4, 1980.
9 Ibid, Aug. 30, 1982.
10 *Salina Journal*, Nov. 4, 1981, History Scrapbook #1, CIHF Archives.
11 *Rope*, Sept. 8, 1980.
12 Ibid, Oct. 6, 1980.

came up. The dragon was tired, really "draggin.'" It turned out that he ate candy and snacks all the time, but not a good breakfast. He was afraid people in ONEderland would laugh at him and was not sure he wanted to go. He was told he must eat better, and that people in this country were not dull. They had fun being healthy and using their energy. They even ate ice cream sometimes, just not all the time.

Other sequences made other points. There was a restaurant scene showing that people usually left the parsley on the plate, perhaps the healthiest thing in their entire meal. Karla the Clown, herself a larger-than-life but graceful African-American woman, read a letter from a girl worried that she is laughed at because she is heavy. Karla, with her positve self-image, sang a song about it:

"I may be big, but I'm light on my feet." Included was the refrain:

> Nobody's perfect
> You know that's true
> But I like who I am
> And I like what I do.
> Light on my feet
> Living is Neat
> Light on my feet
> What a Treat
> Floating along like a Butterfly.

It was holistic medicine to be certain, integrating attitude (you are you and don't want to be like U2Me2, who reported to "his sameness") with diet in a magical mix.[13]

It indeed appealed. By the seventh week 2,000 children from 100 cities had joined the OOAK fun club and many teachers had videotaped the program for class use.[14] The show, according to Riordan, "received more mail at the station than Santa Claus." Over $36,000 in free space was donated by the Wichita Mall to exhibit the set of the show, and there

---

13 Videotaped episodes from "One of a Kind," Mabee Library, CIHF.
14 *Rope*, Dec. 1, 1980.

were applications to Shell and Exxon for sponsorship.[15] By the fall of 1981 workshops were being held at 20 area schools, and 75% of the children there said that they already watched the program.[16] The program, said a teacher at a 1982 workshop "made me realize that there was much more of me inside than I had ever let out." Said another: "It feels so good to listen to creative ideas and to know that somewhere it's possible for 'outrageous' things to be accepted…. Maybe I can hope again!"[17]

The audience felt good about it too. "Dear Dr. Hugh," went one letter. "I would like to have a hug, not a spanking. I have been wathing One of a Kind and I relly love to wath your show. It makes me relly, relly happy inside. I am in 3rd grad." The letter highlights that the shows were about health, not spelling, and the sentiment was clear.[18]

Good local critical response made it unanimous. Bob Curtright of the *Wichita Eagle* liked it, and hoped that it would draw many away from the violent Saturday morning cartoon fare against which it was competing. It was one of the most elaborate local productions ever done, and was marked by the special effects wizardry (1980 style, of course) by Dean Dodson, the creative director of KARD, working with Live Action Video Animation in New York. U2Me2 was a child sized android from the planet Conformus, who learned from the Rainbow Lady about emotions and feelings. His appearance was appealing enough to get his message across. It was a kind of therapy, Riordan said, but "therapy suggests that there is something wrong. No, we are interested in what's right, and promoting that." It was Personal Health Control for Kids.[19]

In 1981 another 13 weekly episodes were produced. "It's probably too far down the road to envision Wichita as a major center for originating children's TV programming," a reporter commented. But the program in a three channel pre-cable town got 21% of the audi-

---

15 Letter, Riordan to Olive Garvey, March 9, 1981, Office Files, CIHF Archives.
16 *Rope*, Oct. 19, 1981.
17 Ibid, Jan. 4, 1982.
18 Ibid, Oct. 11, 1982.
19 Clipping, n.d., in History Scrapbook #1, CIHF Archives.

ence against "Fat Albert" (28%) and NCAA Football (26%). The first series had been purchased for showing in Topeka, Oklahoma City, and Tulsa, there were plans to syndicate it, and broadcasters in Phoenix, Milwaukee, and Houston were giving it a look.[20] It was purchased by the Oklahoma State Department of Education for use in schools.[21] The critics again supported it: "Considering the usual throwaway Saturday morning kiddie fare, 'One of a Kind' continues to be a pleasant change of pace with flashy graphics, quality animation and interesting characters. And it doesn't hurt that it has something substantial (notably nutrition and exercise) behind the fun."[22]

In September 1982, "One of Kind" began a third season. "It doesn't preach," wrote the paper, "and it doesn't nag."[23] It had become very sophisticated as a teaching tool by then, and teachers were sent 13 packets of activity sheets and exercises of the type Riordan had been putting together since the consulting days at "434 Inc." The topics were: "Spaceship Earth," "Listening to Our Bodies and Each Other," "Being Friends to Ourselves and Others," "Building Our Bodies: Relaxation Exercises," "Communicating Ideas, Feelings," "Animal Friends," "Sleep and Dreams," "Healing: Wounds and Feelings," "Say It With Music," "Create, Create, Create," "Understanding Emotions," and "A Positive Self Concept."

There were many suggestions:

> Have the children feel their heartbeats. Explain that the heart beats 70-80 times a minute. Make a stethoscope with a rolled up paper tube and listen to the rhythm of yourself. Squeeze a tennis ball ten times a minute (the normal pulse) to get an idea how the heart works. Then explain that this pumping happens 2.5 billion times in life. If one could slow the heart down through diet and exercise there would be more years

---

20 *Wichita Eagle Beacon,* Feb. 20, 1981, ibid.
21 Clipping, n.d., in History Scrapbook #1, CIHF Archives.
22 *Wichita Eagle Beacon,* Sept. 11, 1981, ibid.
23 Ibid, Sept. 13, 1982.

of vigorous life. Have the children flex their muscles. There are 600 muscles in the body. The average person's muscle exertion daily amounts to the equivalent of loading 24,000 lbs. onto a four ft. high shelf. Have the children make a personal coat of arms. Have them bring five objects that represent their past. Have them develop commercials to "sell" themselves.

Most exercises included a song by Moore Anderson and Myrliss Hershey. The dragon sang: "When your fears start haunting you and you're not sure just what to do. You feel there are no friends, no one around to stop and share. Remember you can shake hands with the dragon. When your spirits are saggin'. Just go up and say hello and it won't take long and you will know that you can meet your fears head on. Each time you do it will make you strong. So step right up and say hello and the dragon of fear will have to go."[24] Another problem was addressed by a piece with the lyric: "Anger, anger I feel it everywhere. Churnin' in my stomach and burnin' neath my hair."

There was of course the "One of a Kind" theme song itself:

> You're one of a kind.
> It's kind of wonderful
> Just how amazing you are.
> Your body and mind
> Are nearly magical,
> Come on and follow your star.
>
> We're all different in some ways
> Yet we're all the same.
> We're alone yet together,
> We're all playing the game
> Of life so . . .

---

[24] "One of a Kind" teacher's work kit in History Scrapbook #1, CIHF Archives.

One of a Kind

You want to be kind
To yourself and stay
Happy and healthy and free
'Cause you're one of a kind,
And that's the best way to be,
That's the best way to be.

The Rainbow on the show was described as a way of viewing life. "The storm and the rainbow, like pain and happiness in life, go hand in hand. What seems painful or 'bad' can become a positive learning experience. The rainbow is a symbol of this integration of experience into a healthy attitude of life."[25]

"One of a Kind" was a big experiment and, locally, it would have to be called a big success. It received national critical recognition, too, winning the silver medal at the New York International Film and TV Festival in 1982 while Dr. Riordan, Frank Chappel, and Myrliss Hershey were in attendance. [26] It was a finalist for the prestigious Iris awards in 1983, where the winner was a series, a single episode of which cost more than the entire "One of a Kind" series. It was nominated that year for a Golden Mike national award by the State of Kansas. In April 1983, it was estimated that 14 million viewers nationwide were seeing it and that 20% of the viewing public had access to it.[27] But it ran its course. For one thing, Riordan notes, it was based on the idea that kids had an attention span of maybe two minutes. Kids surveyed said they liked no pauses, good music, and not too long segments. However, he believed it could run again in the 21st century -- "it's really not that much of a dated show." It did run as #1 in its time slot in New York City for a time and #2 in Philadelphia. At one point, Riordan went to Washington, DC to sign a contract with the Public Broadcasting System to run the program on all their stations. However, that was shortly after the election of Ronald Reagan, whose administration soon

---

25 Clipping, n.d., in ibid.
26 Riordan talk, n.d., [1983], in ibid.
27 *Rope*, March 28, April 4, April 11, April 18, 1983.

eliminated the teeth in the federal mandate that broadcasters had to air some children's programming that was actually good for kids. That did not fit the *laissez-faire* attitude of the new administration, so Riordan found the PBS people in shock at massive cuts. One of the things that had to go was the plan to run "One of a Kind" on public television nationwide. ARAMCO, the US oil conglomerate in Saudia Arabia, used it overseas, and some local PBS stations used it, but as a national phenomenon it was "close, but no cigar."[28]

Still, the program was a near miracle given its production budget, the struggling medical center in Kansas that made it, and the competition. Certainly, it became part of The Center's folklore about what could happen when a few people became very determined and made an attempt to communicate worthwhile values and practices to a public inundated, it was true, with trash, but yearning for something better. It created hope that the other initiatives that would join in the new buildings north of the city would find a home in people's minds and hearts also.

Mrs. Garvey was quiet mostly, not visible much to the staff, never micromanaging, but in constant personal contact with Dr. Riordan about the details of the dream they both shared. She did visit the staff regularly, and maintained a positive rapport with them. Riordan sent her flowers and little gifts on her birthday and Christmas, and they exchanged handwritten notes and letters about The Center.[29] "Your amazing array of lines of expertise," she wrote him, "certainly extends to your taste in exquisite gifts."[30] He sent a crystal bottle, a cloisonné vase and even French bonbons for a once in awhile treat for the chocolate-loving Olive.[31]

Big decisions were made this way. In June 1979, Riordan wrote her that Dr. Hinshaw's part-time consulting arrangement would no longer be practical. A hospital in Ponca City, Oklahoma, had offered him a much higher base pay. Hinshaw had been working for The Center

---

28 Interview, Dr. Hugh Riordan with Craig Miner, June 3, 1998.
29 Letter, Olive Garvey to Dr. Hugh Riordan, Sept. 18, 1979, Office Files, CIHF Archives.
30 Ibid, n.d., [after July 15, 1982].
31 Ibid, Jan. 5, 1983.

for $12,000 a year, and to replace him even with a part-time pathologist would cost perhaps $50,000. Most important, Hinshaw had been with The Center from the beginning and believed in it. In one incident that got into Center folklore, Hinshaw, who had had some doubts about the allergy tests, observed a "lovely, charming, pleasant young woman become totally psychotic and highly combative" within minutes of being given the ingredients in beer and gin to which it had been determined she was sensitive. Dr. Hinshaw and Dr. Riordan had to transport her to the hospital in a semi-restrained state, during which journey Dr. Hinshaw became a strong believer in adverse food reactions. "He has observed first hand over and over again," Riordan wrote, "that what we claim to be true indeed is. To bring another pathologist to the same level of awareness, if he was broad minded, would take at least three years. To have another pathologist with the same level of integrity and competence might be even more difficult." To make him this offer, however, would require more money from Mrs. Garvey for the next two years.[32]

Olive wrote back that she would be glad to support trying to attract Hinshaw. He remained a full time employee at The Center for a time, then established himself in environmental medicine, and, at his retirement in 1998, returned to The Center as a volunteer.

Mrs. Garvey replied to the letters concerning Hinshaw that she hoped The Center would make the most of honors being given to its consultant, Dr. Berry. And she guessed the name change for The Center was OK. "I was reared on the idea that the right hand shouldn't tell what the left hand is doing, which is a bit hard to overcome. And also, it seems to me that your name should be associated with the project." Her advisors, however, had overruled her on that subject, and so Olive W. Garvey Center it was.[33]

Attacks in fact continued, and Riordan needed his supporters sometimes to keep his own spirits up. He wrote Garvey a long letter in

---

[32] Letter, Riordan to Olive Garvey, June 8, 1979, ibid. Interview, Dr. Hugh Riordan with Craig Miner, October 22, 1998.
[33] Letter, Olive Garvey to Riordan, June 12, 1979, Office Files, CIHF Archives.

March 1981 on that theme. He had visited Linus Pauling on his 80th birthday that February and learned that The Center, which had begun to treat cancer patients, was the only place in the world giving intravenous vitamin C to people with terminal cancer. Olive had been urging him to write a book, and that motivated him to think of doing so. He would call it, he said, "Is There Any Hope?" and it would be based on the distance between standard medical thought "entrenched in a huge bureaucracy," and the observations made at The Center. He would document results in migraines, cancer, arthritis, and mental illness. "Unfortunately, as I look back on others who have tried to challenge orthodox medicine it is clear that the book will bring about attack, loss of income from any possible future practice of standard medicine, potential loss of license, and a variety of other inconveniences." Even so, he must continue. "I think we are right or at least more right than other ways currently in practice." He needed to maintain "my own level of personal integrity which includes knowing that I am doing everything possible for my fellow man." He would be talking to Bill Schul about these things, and Bill would help draft the book. That book was never written, nor was one he actually drafted on the computer in 1981 entitled *Burn Him at the Stake and Use Damp Straw*, but eventually in his three volume history called *Medical Mavericks* Riordan did treat the theme, on his mind for obvious reasons, of medicine's trying to destroy its innovators.[34]

Garvey and Riordan also corresponded a great deal about the Master Facility, and about the development of other giving to support it. "Most people," Riordan wrote her, "would rather give to a Harvard or to another big university." Someone had just given $3 million to the University of West Virginia Medical School to endow a chair in nutrition. Riordan commented caustically: "He will have to wait a few years for his disillusionment which might be lessened by an honorary degree." That is to say, it was unlikely that the money would be used as intended. In fact, it was not. So many people told Riordan they wanted to give to a big established institution, and so few could see that those institutions

---

34 Letter, Riordan to Olive Garvey, March 1, 1981, ibid.; *Rope*, March 11, 1982.

at one time started small with a vision. He researched their origins, and found that it was the "sustaining belief" of one or two people that got them going every time. Riordan hoped to gain a critical mass of giving in several areas by 1982 but felt that probably the Master Facility, largely funded by Garvey, would have to exist first. "Each step in our evolution seems to cost more and take two to three more years in time and energy than originally contemplated." The original estimate of $5.5 million for the Master Facility had been pared to $2 million, he wrote her in August 1981, but that was still a great deal of money. [35]

Garvey responded with money and ideas. She thanked Riordan for sending her a model of the Master Facility, commenting that it was "a fitting realization of the alleged purpose of The Center as an avant-garde implementation of natural resources in all things." Her original concept, she told him, was to have a diagnostic lab where anyone and everyone could get a "tailor-made record of his own physical-chemical makeup, and where a knowledgeable staff could supply him with a schedule of his needs to meet his demands for health." The Center had done that, but Garvey was a bit upset that it cost too much to give everyone access. Like Henry Ford, who wanted to manufacture something everyone could enjoy, Olive, in the Garvey family tradition, had a common touch and loved the thought of impacting the daily lives of many, ordinary people. The demand was there, she noted in the fall of 1981. There was a deluge of health and diet books, "but it is a mass response, not an individual response. The quacks are getting rich and the populace is ruining its health with ignorant experimentation."

She had detailed recommendations. The Center did good diagnosis, she thought, but how much "definitive information" did it furnish patients on diet and future regimen? Riordan had once said he could provide a diagnosis that would cost $100. That was Garvey's goal she said, but every day "I see people who need your help, but when I say $500 they groan." The Center had done many good things, but she would like to be sure those included her original purpose at an affordable cost, namely "one person=one tailor-made diagnosis=one diet and regimen."

---

35 Letter, Riordan to Olive Garvey, Aug. 30, 1981, Office Files, CIHF Archives.

Yes, there needed to be more contributors. "I don't believe in monopolies, especially charitable ones." With more people involved, The Center would get more ideas as well as money. "So I had hoped that you could get outside money for your buildings. But, apparently, it is a question of the chicken and the egg. So perhaps the chicken will have to accept responsibility for her offspring."[36]

Riordan responded right away that he thought he could do something for $100, namely a computerized dietary survey, a blood analysis for vitamins ABCE and high density lipoproteins, and a recommendation from a nutritionally aware dietitian.[37] That was the origin of an introductory testing program that continued right to the 21st century, eventually called "Beat the Odds."

It was, Riordan wrote to the Garvey Foundation director after a meeting with Mrs. Garvey, "always a pleasure just to be in her presence." It was, however, not easy to get the money he needed, and even more difficult to get a promise of multi-year support of the kind he thought he needed for planning.[38]

There was the relationship with the rest of the family to consider. Olive's son James, and her daughters Ruth and Olivia did not live in Wichita, but her son Willard did. All became supporters and participants in The Center at various times and in various ways. Each also was an individual with ideas about how things might be done.

Riordan had taken photos of the model under various lighting conditions. He had thought about what the Master Facility would look like on a hot August day and when the moonlight illuminated the pyramid, lake and waterfall.[39] He planted alfalfa to restore the soil.[40] He was concerned too not to disturb what might have been an Indian burial ground on the farm where The Center was to be built, so constructed the underground portions in a berm above the original ground

---

36 Letter, Olive Garvey to Riordan, Sept. 1, 1981, ibid.
37 Letter, Riordan to Olive Garvey, Sept. 7, 1981, ibid.
38 Letter, Riordan to Clifford Allison, Sept. 8, 1981, ibid.
39 Letter, Riordan to Olive Garvey, Oct. 7, 1981, ibid.
40 Interview, Dr. Hugh Riordan and Craig Miner, October 22, 1998.

level. He was thinking of the dynamic tension in the geodesic domes and the organic shapes and the conservation of energy. To him each dome would sound and feel different depending on how many "penetrations" it had, and each would operate differently as an environment for staff and patients. About 40 inches down in the ground at the site there was a layer of quartzite about 1/4 inch thick which, Riordan said later, had "something to do with the energy of this place." He looked for water using water witches. He worried about the fertilizer and insecticides that had been used on the farm, and that there was not a worm detected in test borings within two feet of the surface when construction started.[41]

Willard Garvey, who for years was president of Builders, Inc., definitely had advice on the building. "I must admit," Riordan wrote to Willard's mother, "to a great deal of trepidation over the new building, not from a management standpoint when completed but because I am concerned that Willard's unique perspective of how things should be done might prevail. I am sure that he is extremely able to bring in projects for a minimum cost …. In the long run, however, I am not sure that for us some expected construction economies would really pay off."

Riordan wanted his structure to last 100 years. "I really do not want leaking floors, walls or roofs interfering with our capacity to devote full attention to work." Landscaping might seem a frill "but if we are going to influence people to make The Center the recipient of donations we should have aesthetically pleasing grounds at least at the entrance and the area surrounding. "I think," Riordan wrote, "that if this Master Facility is built it should be a monument not to the architect but to the degree of excellence that we try to maintain at The Olive W. Garvey Center for the Improvement of Human Functioning, to your personal vision and inspiration and to the Garvey name."[42]

The continuing exchanges between Riordan and Olive were quite personal. The relationship of the two was growing closer. "My arm is much better," Olive wrote Hugh in November 1981. She had been driv-

---

41 Ibid, May 27, 1998.
42 Letter, Riordan to Olive Garvey, Oct. 7, 1981, Office Files, CIHF Archives.

ing her car that week. "I wish you could give me a little strength and energy as I feel a lack of both. Or is it just my *age*?" She was taking some B15 though she had heard it was controversial. The dosage was six a day, but she was taking only three. However, she knew, she said, that Dr. Riordan would not send them to her unless he considered them safe.[43] Later she wrote: "I suppose confession is good for the soul, so I must confess that maybe I have been a bit negligent of my health." On Christmas day, 1982, her teeth began getting sore, became infected, and required a root canal operation. That left her weak. And the holidays were hard on her nutritionally. She remembered having ham hocks and beans for dinner one night and corned beef hash for breakfast. That sent her blood pressure to 190 over 92. "My children do not serve my accustomed menus," she said, and recalled one other time when she had measured high blood pressure after eating a salty snack.[44] In 1982, Riordan began to treat other members of the family as well.[45]

She confided to Riordan about her reading. In 1983, she was reading Jess Stern's book about Taylor Caldwell under hypnosis (*Search for a Soul* [1974]). Caldwell had recalled a life as an instructor in a medical school in Athens in the time of Pericles. There she gave a lecture covering all the principles of holistic medicine, as well as the discovery of penicillin. "It is fantastic," Garvey wrote Dr. Riordan.[46]

She also wrote him regularly about her own spiritual experiences, and those of a friend, who was something of a medium. In the spring of 1983, as construction was beginning on the Master Facility, Riordan wrote that he had heard from a spiritual healer in California who said that in 1972 a spirit had conveyed to her the shape of a healing center which should be built. He enclosed a copy of her design sketch done 11 years earlier and containing many elements of the CIHF campus. "I find it rather mind blowing."[47] She responded that it was amazing -- "the only devia-

---

[43] Letter, Olive Garvey to Riordan, Nov. 26, 1981, ibid.
[44] Ibid, Jan. 5, 1983.
[45] Letter, Riordan to Olive Garvey, Jan. 31, 1982, ibid.
[46] Letter, Olive Garvey to Riordan, April 4, 1983, ibid.
[47] Letter, Riordan to Olive Garvey, June 17, 1983, ibid.

tion is the location and exact shape of the pyramid." Aline, her spiritualist friend, told her that "everything is planned in cosmic and its realization on earth depends on someone being able to realize the idea, plan or image. Everything 'happens' there, first. However everything foreseen does not necessarily 'realize' as earthlings still have a 'choice.'" Aline had frequently had messages from the spirit world about The Center and "they" mostly approved. Olive, however, was skeptical enough to ask Hugh if he had checked the authenticity of the date of the plan, and whether the psychic had seen a plan of the CIHF campus. She thanked him for advice on liquids in the same letter, and promised to cut down on coffee.[48]

While the buildings on North Hillside were slowly developing — a long time, it seemed in planning, and too long in construction — the staff developed, the international conferences continued, and, of course, more and more patients were helped.

Marilyn Landreth arrived in December 1977, as a student extern from the WSU Department of Psychology.[49] She remained for her 20-year pin and beyond. Mavis Schultz began as a nurse in 1977 and was still a nurse at The Center in 2000. She went back to school while at The Center and went through the nurse-clinician program.[50] Landreth and Catherine Willner began in the spring of 1979 to call voluntary bimonthly one-hour-long meetings of employees concerning their work functions, personal experiences, philosophy, and directions.[51] Willner went on to become a neurologist after training at the Mayo Clinic. Also in 1979, the Junior League of Wichita placed a volunteer at The Center.[52] Jo Carpenter took over supervision of the lab.[53] Sharon Neathery was working at the Bio Center lab then, "bringing with her her nursing baby who seems to enjoy the environment there."[54] Neathery was one of four mothers who brought their nursing babies to The Center at that time, an unusual

---

48 Letter, Olive Garvey to Riordan, June 20, 1983, ibid.
49 *Rope*, Dec. 12, 1977.
50 Staff Profiles, Mabee Library, CIHF.
51 Ibid, n.d., [Spring, 1979].
52 Ibid, April 2, 1979.
53 *Rope*, Feb. 5, 1979.
54 Ibid, April 30, 1979.

practice in businesses then. It fitted the holistic philosophy to assume that employees had lives outside their work. In 1980 Donna Kramme answered an ad about a need of The Center for a word processor, and at the dawn of the 21st century, she was still working there.[55] Kramme remembered later that she thought at first the place was crazy: the lady who interviewed her had an intravenous drip in her arm and Donna wondered if they were into drugs. She soon learned, however, saw results with patients, and was active in everything from blowing up balloons for the Skybreakings to organizing the fan club for "One of a Kind."[56] In 1981, Maurice Johnson, a former IRS district director, joined to help Laura Benson computerize some of the controls and accounting.[57] An extra attraction with him was his wife of forty years, Betty, who had a degree in Home Economics from Kansas State University and had worked on the AT-10 project at Beechcraft during World War II. She had returned to WSU for a degree in Anthropology and volunteered in The Center library.[58] Oscar Rasmussen, PhD worked in the lab 10 days a month on clinical research.[59] 1982 brought Farhad Tadayon, a mechanical engineer who had done biofeedback research; Bruce Underwood, who worked part-time with The Center as PHC coordinator and part with the Kansas Cardiology Associates PA as an exercise physiologist and later full-time at The Center; John Nguyen, an East High student computer whiz who had topped two million points in the video game Pac Man and scored 780 of 800 on his SAT test in math.[60] Nguyen wrote the computer lab program which was used for a number of years and eventually got a PhD at MIT. Some came and went (development directors and fiscal administrators especially often) and some stayed to get their 20-year pins (Shultz, Benson, Neathery, Kramme, Landreth), but for all, working at The Center was an unforgettable, unique experience. For the most part, too, their specific assignments changed as they did.

---

55 Staff Profiles, Mabee Library, CIHF.
56 Interview, Donna Kramme with Craig Miner, October 29, 1998.
57 *Rope*, March 11, 1982.
58 Staff Profiles, Mabee Library, CIHF.
59 *Rope*, March 11, 1982.
60 Ibid, Aug. 16, 1982. *Wichita Eagle Beacon*, n.d. 1982, History Scrapbook #1.

One of a Kind

Not all employees worked out. One was a physician who was hired with good credentials and high interest in nutrition. Shortly after he started, Dr. Riordan was out of town for a couple of days and upon his return the nurses asked him if he knew how the new doctor was taking calls. He said 'no,' and they told him that they had to drive out to his house and give him his messages because he did not have a telephone. Dr. Riordan left a note for him, saying if he was having trouble getting a phone to let him know because he could get it taken care of right away. The response to the note was, that the doctor did not wish to have a telephone. He was terminated within two weeks. Upon reflection, Dr. Riordan said that it was not a part of the job interview up to that time to ask a physician if he/she would mind having a telephone.

Consultants associated in flocks, it sometimes seemed. Dr. Catherine Spears signed on as a consultant early in 1978.[61] Spears's mother was a psychiatric nurse and her father a CPA. Catherine was born in Brooklyn, always wanted to be a doctor, and got her degree while working in the daytime as a secretary in the legal department of an insurance company. She was a great success, as she could translate documents into Swedish, French or German. She came to specialize in handicapped children in her pediatric practice and believed "that she could not effectively help handicapped children until she first understood normal ones both sick and well." She first met Riordan when they attended a Chinese medicine conference in 1973 and then again when both studied auricular therapy with Dr. Paul Nogier in Lyons, France.[62] She would come to The Center from New Jersey and see children with cerebral palsy and eye problems. She once did a local TV series on crossed eyes and ways to cure them without surgery, which enraged at least one local pediatric ophthalmologist, but worked. She later had several surgeries that made it almost impossible for her even to sit for any period, but she continued her work. The Center insisted on paying her, but she would donate all of it back because of her support for The

---

61 *Rope*, Jan. 18, 1978. Interview, Dr. Hugh Riordan with Craig Miner, February 1, 2000.
62 Staff Profiles, Mabee Library, CIHF.

Center's mission.[63] There were pictures on the stairs down to the Taste of Health restaurant in the Marge Page Dome of some of the giants behind The Center. One of them was a thin redheaded woman with no identifying label. That was Catherine Spears. "It feels a little funny calling such a great lady by her first name," an employee said. But that is the way things were done at the Garvey Center.[64]

Dr. Charles Berry, MD, MPH, former chief of Aerospace Medicine for NASA, joined as consultant for Personal Health Control in 1979, was active in the "One of a Kind" project, and contributed to the classes at Friends University titled the Physiology and Psychology of Fatigue and Personal Health Control. Berry received the American Medical Association's highest award in 1979 and was nominated for the Nobel prize in Medicine.[65] Russ Jaffe MD, PhD, who worked with the National Institutes of Health for years, visited in 1979 as a consultant to test a new way to do the cytotoxic test.[66]

In 1980, Riordan met Philip Callahan, PhD in Gainesville, Florida, where Callahan was a biologist for the US Department of Agriculture. He had manned a secret radio station in Ireland in World War II and earned his doctorate at Kansas State University. He was interested in infrared communication among insects and animals. He wrote numerous books on the topic, including *Insect Behavior, Insects and How They Function, The Evolution of Insects, Tuning into Nature,* and *Bird Behavior,* as well as children's books and an autobiography called *Ghost Moth.* He had even hitchhiked around the world.[67] Riordan thought he was a true genius, invited him to the 4th International Conference, and began a consulting relationship with him. His first job was to do infrared research, and his only pay at first was for his expenses.[68]

Dr. Myrliss Hershey and others came on board in 1980 mostly for

---

63 Interview, Dr. Hugh Riordan with Craig Miner, June 10, 1998.
64 Staff Profiles, Mabee Library, CIHF.
65 *Rope,* June 11, 1979.
66 Ibid, June 25, 1979.
67 Staff Profiles, Mabee Library, CIHF. Interview, Dr. Hugh Riordan with Craig Miner, October 22, 1998.
68 *Rope,* March 17, 1980.

One of a Kind

the TV production.[69] By 1981 consultants included Vic Eichler, PhD in biological research; Dr H. Doubler in auricular medicine; Dr. David Kleier in internal medicine; Dwight Krehbiel, PhD in physiologic psychology; Rod Sobieski, PhD in microbiology; and A. Wayne Wiens, PhD in genetic biochemistry.[70] Bruce Burr, a student at Bethel College at the time, worked with The Center and later became an MD. Space was so tight that it used to be said that the first one there in the morning got the chair.[71] While such a crew led to warnings from Olive Garvey that the staff was getting too big too fast and Riordan was spreading himself too thin, he commented that such prestigious consultants were most helpful for the public reputation as well as for the scientific work of The Center, as people realized that prominent figures did not associate their names with an institution unless they were confident of its work.[72]

Part of the attraction both for staff and consultants was Riordan himself, and part of it was the atmosphere at The Center -- intense, yet non-bureaucratic, open and personal. Riordan always told the employees that if they could not get to work he would pick them up himself. Once on a snowy day, Riordan loaded the staff who had braved the elements into his blue Mercury and treated them to lunch. On the way back the windows were steamed up from the crowded car, he rolled down the window a bit and slush splattered on his head and his eyelids. Everyone barely contained their mirth, but there was a silence until Riordan himself laughed and then there was an explosion.[73] When one of the staff had back problems and got an estimate from a chiropractor for $1,892 in treatments, including traction therapy, ultra sound and diathermy, Riordan did auricular therapy for free and fixed the problem. Even had the person not been an employee and gotten the care

---

69 Ibid, Aug. 4, 1980.
70 Ibid, Jan. 5, 1981.
71 Interview, Marilyn Landreth with Craig Miner, Aug. 18, 1999.
72 *Rope*, Jan. 28, 1980.
73 Interview, Marilyn Landreth and Laura Benson with Craig Miner, Aug. 18, 1999.

free, the fee for the acupuncture would have been only $260.[74] The Center staff had holiday dinners together.[75] The extra half hour at lunch encouraged interaction, exercise, reflection, or, in short, doing something entirely different from the ordinary fare during this period.[76] In 1981, a mimeographed employee newsletter, called *Human News* was started.[77] Employees were recognized for service with at least a lunch. Laura Benson, The Center's second such employee, received her recognition in April 1981, just after Riordan got back from a study tour in France lining up speakers for the 6th International Conference.[78] Those things created longevity in staff, since most felt "they're well respected and have a role to play." It cost $30,000 to replace an employee and get a new one up to speed, but it was not just the bottom line that motivated the policy. Just as cutting to the bone on construction costs was not, to Riordan, healthy, neither was eliminating the flowers, the dinners and lunches and sometimes even the trips together for the staff. The perks and the chance to work in any field where needed ("very few people here do what they are supposed to") all contributed to productivity and creativity, Riordan thought, and those were what made the staff worth having.[79] Many staff people said they wanted to work at The Center because people there were not afraid to be "on the point." Arline Magnusson, for example, a nurse volunteer, wrote that "after three kids, two marriages, life in nine states and a progressively successful career in the Veteran's Administration, I started to look for competence in promotion of health, mine and others, rather than just in patching up illnesses, big and small."[80] Jan Metz, herself described by one of her fellows as "like a river, rushing and swirling," was hired as a receptionist. She liked Riordan, she said, because of his breadth of vision and thinking, his phi-

---

74 *Rope*, Nov. 10,. 1980.
75 Ibid, Dec. 1, 1980.
76 Interview, Dr. Hugh Riordan with Craig Miner, June 10, 1998.
77 *Rope*, Sept. 24, 1981.
78 Ibid, April 27, 1981.
79 Interview, Dr. Hugh Riordan with Craig Miner, June 10, 1998.
80 Staff Profiles, Mabee Library, CIHF.

losophies, his free-thinking, open ideas."[81] Riordan's reaction to all this was: "Of course, it is very exciting, rewarding and somewhat frustrating to be 'on the point.' But it is the only place for us to be." [82]

Many younger doctors who developed prestigious reputations later were eternally grateful to The Center for respecting them, listening to them, and giving them either a forum for their ideas or a place for their experiments or both at a time when they were literally being laughed at by quite a few others. There were also older doctors who, like Riordan himself, had spent a career in partial frustration at not being able to help people more, and who perhaps in retirement could start a second career with The Center trying the things they had always wanted to try but couldn't afford to psychologically or financially. The depth of their commitment was shown in their willingness to go to bat for The Center in many ways, from the insurance wars to the various grant applications that were tried for funding the Master Facility.

Dr. Berry, for instance, wrote a letter of support to the Kresge Foundation in 1982, from which The Center had requested $4 million as early as 1979.[83] Riordan had met him by telephone at the suggestion of a mutual friend and they were kindred souls right away. Berry spoke at the 3rd International Conference in 1979 and was a supporter from then on.[84] "I was deeply privileged," he wrote, "to be given the medical responsibility to get man into space and have him return safely.... It was the ultimate experience in preventative medicine." Among the lessons were 1) that healthy people can adapt to abnormal environs, 2) each person is unique and it is necessary to determine individual normal values, 3) "personal commitment is necessary to modify individual lifestyle to meet the demands of mission preparation and accomplishment," and 4) "you must have the courage to act prudently using the information available to progress toward the goal even though you do not have all facts or data." Those were exactly the tenents of The Center. The nation

---

81 Staff Profiles, Mabee Library, CIHF.
82 *Rope*, June 8, 1981.
83 Ibid, April 2, 1979.
84 Staff Profiles, Mabee Library, CIHF.

was in a health care crisis, with costs of 10% of the gross national product and rising. The greatest hope to deal with that was preventative medicine and the promotion of health, exactly what the Olive W. Garvey Center was doing. "I have been asked why I travel from Houston to Wichita each month to consult with this Center when I am engaged in so many activities in the vast Houston medical arena and also nationally. It is simple to state -- it's because the people of this Center are devoted to the cause I have pledged myself to -- the development of a healthier society with more individuals functioning at their optimum capacity -- and they are making it happen. I want to work with them for we stimulate each other."[85] At the time of that letter Berry spoke to the Wichita Downtown Rotary, a group of 500 prominent local business people, who certainly got a new sort of message.[86]

Another letter to the Kresge Foundation came from Dr. Emanuel Cheraskin, MD, DMD. He reemphasized that "while 'sickness' is a booming business, 'health' is the fastest growing failing business in America." Cheraskin had written 500 papers and 13 books to try to "ferret out the fundamentals of true primary prevention," and found the Olive Garvey Center to have the greatest promise in the nation "as a think tank and practical application center."[87]

The conferences continued to draw attention. Dr. Burkitt, 68, was back in 1979 with his heaping teaspoon of bran recommendation.[88] Dr. George Williams, a pathologist, spoke on "Preventative Maintenance of the Health of Industrial Manpower." He documented that 25% of hospital patients were admitted because of depression and/or alcoholism. Backaches cost $1 billion annually and cost $25 billion in lost work time. Pre-employment physical exams only discovered existing conditions: they did nothing to prevent disease. Denis Shapiro, PhD, president of the Institute for the Advancement of Human Behavior and a psycholo-

---

85 Letter of Dr. Charles Berry to Kresge Foundation, Feb. 11, 1982, in Rope, Feb. 22, 1982.
86 *Rope*, Feb. 8, 1982.
87 Letter, Emanuel Cheraskin to Kresge Foundation, Feb. 16, 1982 in Rope, Feb. 22, 1982.
88 *Wichita Eagle*, Sept. 19, 1979, History Scrapbook #1, CIHF Archives.

gist with the Stanford Medical School, spoke on "Self Control: East and West, an Overview." There was an address by Dr. Arlene Putt on biofeedback and stress, and one by Dr. Robert Burns, DDS suggesting that proper diet could prevent 90% of dental diseases. Dr. Berry exclaimed in his speech that, "we need to know more about exercise, nutrition and smoking, but, we already know enough about these to do something."[89]

In September 1980, at the fourth conference, Dr. Steven Halpern opened with his "anti frantic music." Sounds, he said, had great physiological and psychological effects. They could cause irritability, but also ulcers and other stress-related conditions such as heart attacks and migraine headaches. Bad sounds could decrease muscle tone and sap energy. Yet most people were unaware of the sounds that were around them all the time. They had been conditioned to think the roar of an engine was good, as were certain kinds of music, which, according to Halpern, should be on the Surgeon General's list of things dangerous to your health. Just as smoking in public places was restricted, so should sounds from other places. Restaurant music needed turning down, and such music as there was needed be better adapted to the human organism. Halpern called his own compositions "bio music," and claimed they incorporated human harmonics. His talk attracted a crowd, and his book *Tuning the Human Instrument* drew interest in town that fall. "Give the body a chance, " Halpern said, "and it chooses right. The body is like a tuning fork. It already knows the score. It's built in."[90]

Registration was 330 people.[91] There was evidence that these were not just The Center's conferences anymore. The Wichita Sunday paper thought that the fitness "fad" would continue. Ten years ago, if one saw a person running down the street, one might think he was robbing a bank. Now joggers were common. Dr. Robert Fowler, a Wichita cardiologist, ran the Boston Marathon in 1978 and was arguing that jogging fought depression. The enthusiasm for fitness, the paper noted, "has been almost

---

89 Report on 3rd International Conference in *The ACA Journal of Chiropractic* in Rope, Jan, 1980.
90 *Wichita Beacon*, Sept. 17, 1980, ibid.
91 *Rope*, Sept. 8, 1980.

evangelical."[92] An article in the national journal *Nurse Practitioner* in 1981 mentioned The Center and included a chart of money saved through lifestyle changes.[93] *Runner's World* the next summer even contained an article supporting cytotoxic testing of the type The Center did, and claiming that many runners had been helped by discovery of their food allergies.[94]

The 4th International Conference drew together another impressive group. Dr. James Anderson, the chief of the Endocrine-Metabolic section and professor of medicine and clinical nutrition at the University of Kentucky, Lexington, spoke on "Plant Fiber: Dietary Effects on Glucose and Lipid Metabolism." He was not as colorful as Burkitt, but the message was the same. Nedra Belloc, MA, adjunct professor at Southern Oregon State College, spoke on "Recent International Seminar on Biological and Social Aspects of Mortality and Longevity." Dr. Michael Bircheron, a rheumatologist and researcher for the French government, spoke on "A New Intervention for Smoking Cessation." Dr. Phillip Callahan's talk, "Non-Linear Infrared Radiation in Biological Systems with Special Reference to Future Medical Application," lacked a zippy title but had deep content. Dr. Spears spoke on "New Dimensions in the Diagnosis and Treatment of Learning Disabilities." And those were only some highlights. Doctors could attend the three-day conference for $150, other health professionals were $75, and students $15. One could get 15 credit hours of category one credit from the Kansas Dental Board Panel on Continuing Education, the American Dietetic Association, the American Osteopathic Association, or The Center for Continuing Health Education at Wichita State University.[95]

The 5th International Conference in 1981 included the return of many of the regulars and some additions. Registration was more than 400.[96] There were Dr. Norman Childers on "Arthritis and Night-

---

92 *Wichita Eagle and Beacon*, Jan. 27, 1980, ibid.
93 Elizabeth Dayani, Judith Tullock, Patrician M. Huber, "Financing Health Promotion/Wellness," *Nurse Practitioner* (July/August, 1981): 37-38, 41.
94 *Runner's World* (July, 1981): 69-63.
95 Program and Faculty List, 4th International Conference on Human Functioning, Sept. 12-14, 1980, ibid.
96 *Rope*, Sept. 14, 1981.

shades;" B. Robert Crago, PhD on "The Treatment of Chronic Pain: Patient-Therapist Viewpoints;" Effie Poy Yew Chow, RN, PhD, the president of the East-West Academy for Healing Arts, on "Healing Energy Systems: Utilization for Health;" Dr. Robert Hudson, professor of the history and philosophy of medicine at the University of Kansas School of Medicine in Kansas City, whose speech title was "Prima non Nocere: The Case for Restraint in Medical Intervention;" Dr. Theodore Reiff, director of the Institute of Gerontology and Geriatric Medicine at the University of North Dakota on "Overview of Human Aging," and Dr. Jean Jaque Legros of Liege, Belgium, speaking on "Vasopressin and Memory in the Human." Dr. Spears spoke on "Non-Surgical Approach to the Diagnosis and Treatment of Strabismus, and Dr. Pfeiffer on "Useful Micronutrients in the Eighties."[97] One speaker that year was Marilyn Ferguson, editor of the *Brain/Mind Bulletin*, and author of a popular book entitled *The Aquarian Conspiracy*.[98]

Certainly the conferences combated what the newsletter of the Huxley Institute of Canada called, tongue in cheek, the "intransigent Orthodoxy disorder." It had, the newsletter averred, "plagued humans for many centuries, was very difficult to classify because information about it is hard to obtain and objective tests were very difficult to set up because of opposition and even hostility from the subjects." But symptoms definitely included hostility to new ideas and concepts, and "anger, agitation, and even depression when confronted with a new situation or idea. Mainly characterized by irrational opposition to the introduction of new concepts without regard to their value or proven benefits." The disorder quickly reached the chronic stage, was not subject to treatment, and, in most cases, "it has to be considered terminal."[99]

"Thanks a lot," wrote Dr. Karl-Ludvig Reichert from Norway, "for inviting me to your very unique and lovable meeting. You are by your daring and frontier transcending policy indeed breaking 'new paths' in the

---

97 Ibid, April 27, 1981, preliminary list.
98 *Rope*, June 6, 1981.
99 Quoted in Ibid, July 20, 1981.

best American frontier tradition. I found Wichita and you all so humane and lovable that I can only regret 'that to depart is to die a little.'"[100]

Naturally, the group of offices scattered about East Wichita were becoming quite overloaded by 1981, and eagerness for the completion of the Master Facility, for which a construction contact was signed that year, was high.[101] Luckily, no one knew that there would be three celebrations on Mrs. Garvey's July birthday before construction got underway in real earnest and that the move would not take place until 1984. However and wherever, patients remained at The Center, and successes there provided encouragement that banished most of the architect and contractor-generated gloom.

All along, it must be remembered, the central business of The Center was serving patients and co-learners. Case summaries of people who came to The Center are always fascinating.

In 1978 a woman in her thirties called Dr. Riordan for another opinion prior to scheduled bowel surgery. He saw her as part of a group of free evaluations The Center did for people with ileitis and Crohn's disease. She had the latter, which included severe abdominal cramping, bloating, nausea and infrequent large bowel movements. Her Center tests showed she had marked food sensitivities and a severe deficiency of vitamin C. The Center suggested dietary adjustments and therapeutic levels of chelated ascorbates. In several days her elimination was normal and she felt better. A few days after that she reported she had more ambition. She had stopped taking prednisone, a form of cortisone, and the moon face effect of that was lessoned. She stopped taking pain pills, which she had been on for the past year -- not only orally but often injections of Demerol (a narcotic) and Compazine (a tranquilizer). She was accustomed to go to bed at 9 pm utterly exhausted, but after The Center treatment she had much more energy. Everyone noticed the change in her appearance, from looking near dead to looking healthy. She signed up for an aerobic dancing class.[102]

---

100 Ibid, Oct. 26, 1981.
101 Ibid, Oct. 26, 1981. The contract was signed on October 16.
102 Ibid, Aug. 28, 1978.

One of a Kind

About that time, Riordan toyed with the idea of having an association of physicians, particularly family physicians, who would come to The Center for training, and then take some of these techniques back to their regular practice. When there were several in the Wichita area, he could offer stipends to medical students throughout the US to come to study for one week to one month, paying their travel and lodging.[103] It was one of hundreds of ideas he could not implement.

In 1979, the Olive Garvey Center treated a potter who was very ill. He had a high platelet count and there was concern he had leukemia. However, a bone marrow biopsy did not confirm that. But tests showed a zero level of plasma vitamin C, suggesting chronic stress combined with an inadequate C intake. He received injections which lowered his platelet count, but when he changed to oral C his count went up again. The hospital lab showed no heavy metals, but metal contamination was so typical of his symptoms that The Center did chelation on him, and lots of lead and cadmium came out in his urine. Going into his history, the doctors learned that he had used a uranium glaze for the yellow color on his pots. He was told it was not radioactive. The Center had a sample tested. True, there was no gamma radiation, but there was so much beta radiation that the sample was confiscated by governmental authorities. He had been exposed to it for many years. The new equipment required to treat him cost $1,000, but he had little money. The Center treated him anyway and in return he provided pottery (not yellow) for the new Master Facility.[104]

A 1980 Center case made *Newsweek* magazine. A mother wrote that publication that she had struggled over ten years with a hyperactive child, whom she did not want on Ritalin. Finally she found a doctor in Wichita (Riordan), who found that the boy was allergic to chocolate, oatmeal and eggs. There was a vast improvement in a week. "During this past year and a half, we have found that we have a son who is well adjusted, well behaved and a joy to live with. He was not happy with the way he acted -- he could not help himself. In his own words, 'I felt

---

103 Ibid, Oct. 9, 1978.
104 Ibid, Sept. 4, 1979.

all the time like I wanted to explode inside." That kind of case, Riordan commented, was a great reward: "We look forward to being able to do even more in the future," he wrote the mother, "and to make sure that what we know to be true will move from being medical heresy today to medical policy tomorrow."[105]

That same year The Center heard from its first cancer patient, a year after her initial evaluation. Her diagnosis following abdominal surgery had been that the cancer was so scattered that neither surgery nor x-ray would help. The Center therapy included high dose intravenous vitamin C, enzymes, high doses of vitamin A and visualization exercises on how the cancer could be conquered. "Her quality of life so greatly improved after the first weeks of therapy that regardless of the final outcome, her treatment must be regarded as a significant success." She lived much longer than anyone expected.[106]

To a patient who arrived in 1981 Riordan explained that The Center was concerned with the underlying causes of chronic ailments. If a person had a kidney stone, the hospital could remove it. But it gave little attention to the cause or preventing more from forming. "We want to discover why it started when it did instead of the next week, the day before, or the previous month." It was not enough to medicate to cover symptoms. "We view each symptom as the body trying to tell us that something is not quite right. What those symptoms are and how they develop help to provide all important clues in the detective work of finding underlying causes."[107]

People appreciated that kind of innovation, and the willingness to apply the results to them. In 1982, The Center had 11 service areas: Clinical Services, Basic Research Services, Clinical Research Services, Bio Center Laboratory, Biomedical Synergistics Institute, Informational Services, Personal Health Control, Predictive Health Systems, One of a Kind, Health Coach (a telephone advice service), and The

---

105 Ibid, June 30, 1980.
106 Ibid, Nov. 10, 1980.
107 Ibid, Feb. 23, 1981.

One of a Kind

Society for the Improvement of Human Functioning.[108] The Society, which organized public supporters of The Center (now willing to give their names), had 124 members in February 1982, 300 in August of that year, and over 500 by May 1983.[109] The divisions, Riordan wrote, "now form the basic matrix for everything we expect to be able to do in the future." Together, they provided "a synergistic cross fertilization, unique in the scientific world, which allows us to pursue with a broad spectrum view our missions of medical diagnosis, treatment, education, motivation, and research." The Center had seen patients from 46 states and six countries since it started. The Bio Center lab had performed 20,312 tests in the last year and could detect 17 trace elements in urine, 14 in blood and 16 in hair. The operating budget was near $2 million. "At this point in time," went the annual report to supporters, "we know of no other organization of people in the world that offers the logical, interrelated, broad spectrum of services found at the Olive W. Garvey Center for the Improvement of Human Functioning."[110]

Patients agreed at least that something was happening that had not happened before. "For years," one wrote, "I have felt like I was down in a well trying to get out but helpless to do so. It wasn't that people didn't know I was there. They seemed to just look over the edge, peer down and say 'Get out of there!' But no one would throw me a rope. Thanks to you at The Center for throwing me a rope and helping me climb out to have a satisfying life."[111] From that story the name of The Center's letter to its donors had come. Said another, a 67 year-old veteran of 680 doses of antibiotics without result before coming to The Center: "I feel like I've joined the living again."[112]

---

108 Ibid, March 11, 1982.
109 Ibid, Feb. 8, Aug. 23, 1982, May 27, 1983.
110 Ibid, March 11, 1982.
111 Ibid, Aug. 10, 1981.
112 Ibid, July 19, 1982.

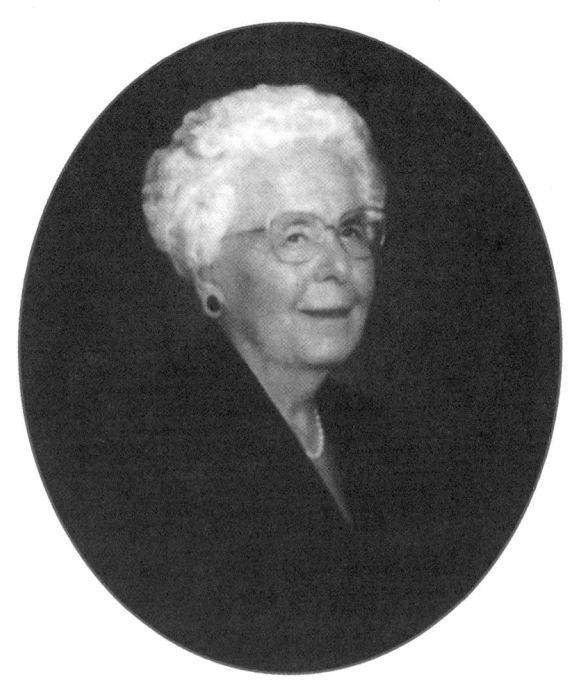

OLIVE WHITE GARVEY
1893-1993

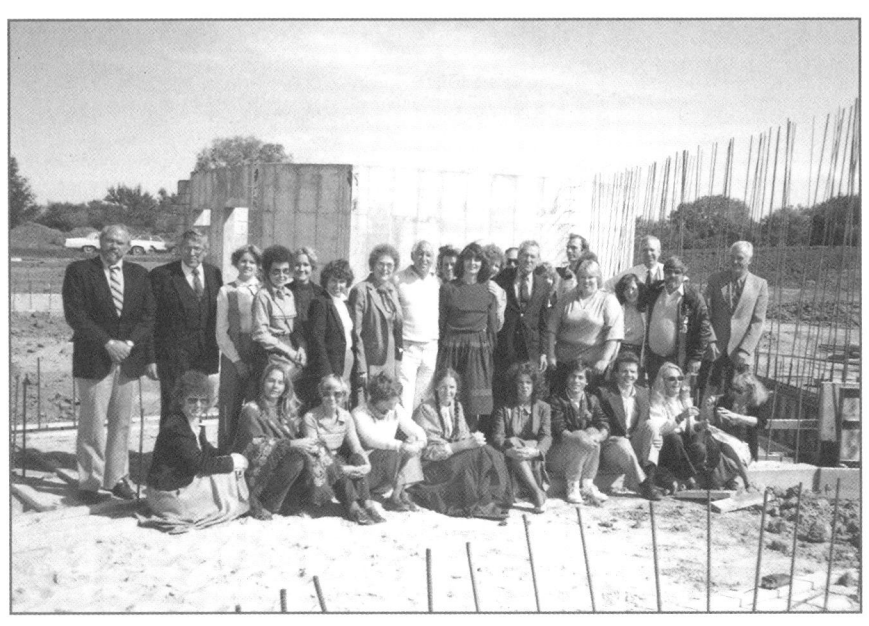

Construction starts with many problems ahead.

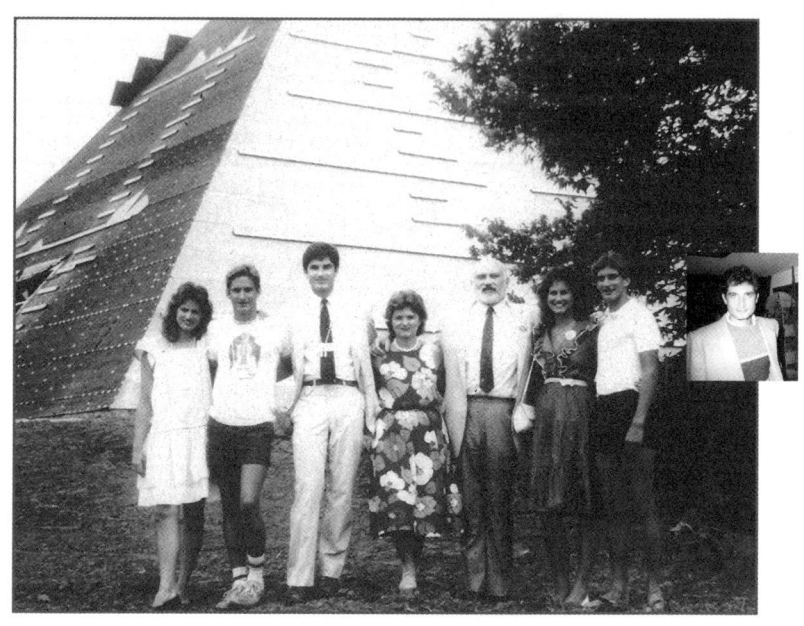

RIORDAN FAMILY
Left to Right: Teresa, Brian, Michael, Jan, Hugh, Renee, Quinn and Neil.

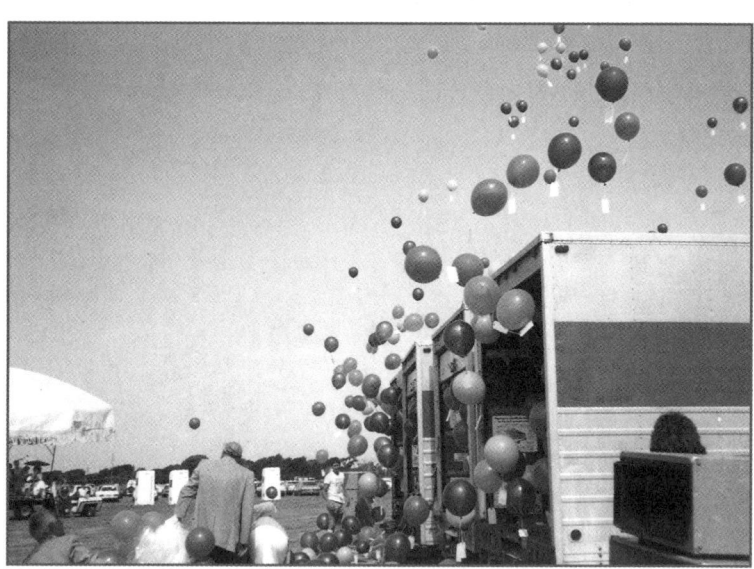

THEY'RE OFF!
Skybreaking at the Master Facility July, 1983.

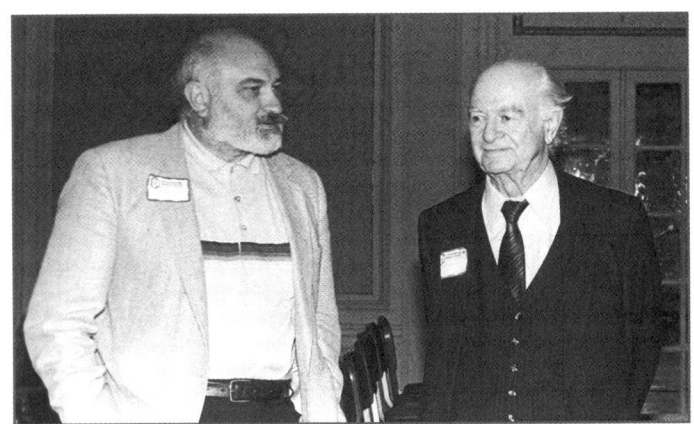

Hugh Riordan with Linus Pauling, who was famous for his Vitamin C research.

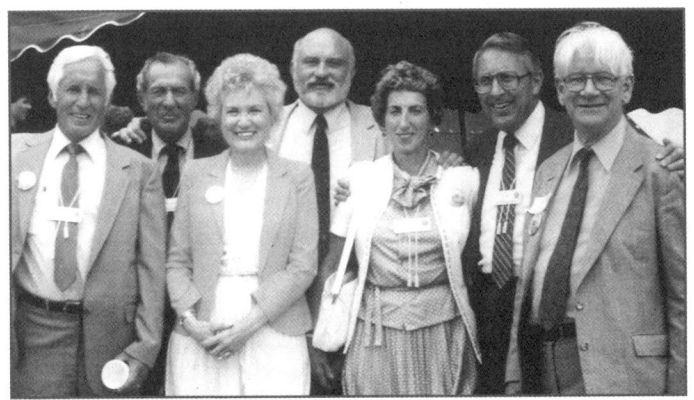

EARLY PIONEERS OF THE CENTER
Left to Right: Bill Schul PhD, Emanual Cheraskin MD, Myellis Hershey PhD, Hugh Riordan MD, Catherine Spears MD, Chuck Berry MD and Carl Pfeiffer PhD.

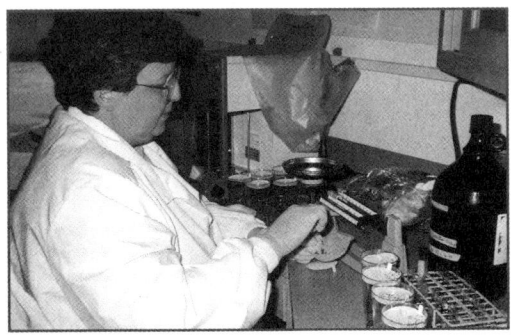

Sharon Neathery testing in lab.

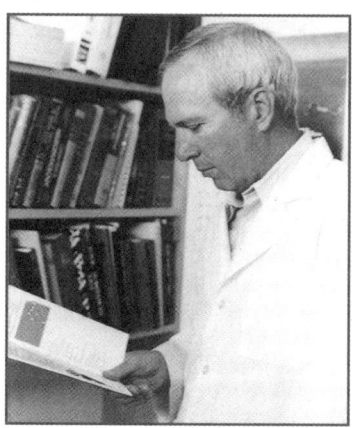

Pahologist Charles Hinshaw MD in Mabee Library.

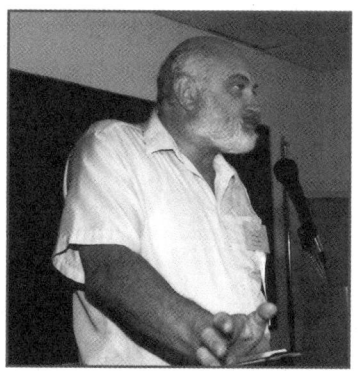

Riordan presiding at Center's Second International Congress, Sept. 1978.

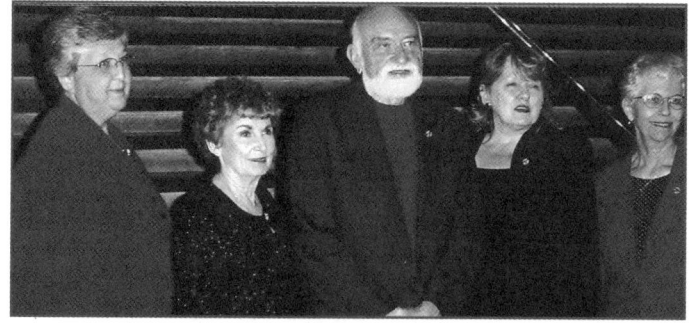

FOUNDING EMPLOYEES
Left to Right: Sharon Neathery, Marilyn Landreth, Hugh Riordan, Laura Benson & Mavis Schultz.

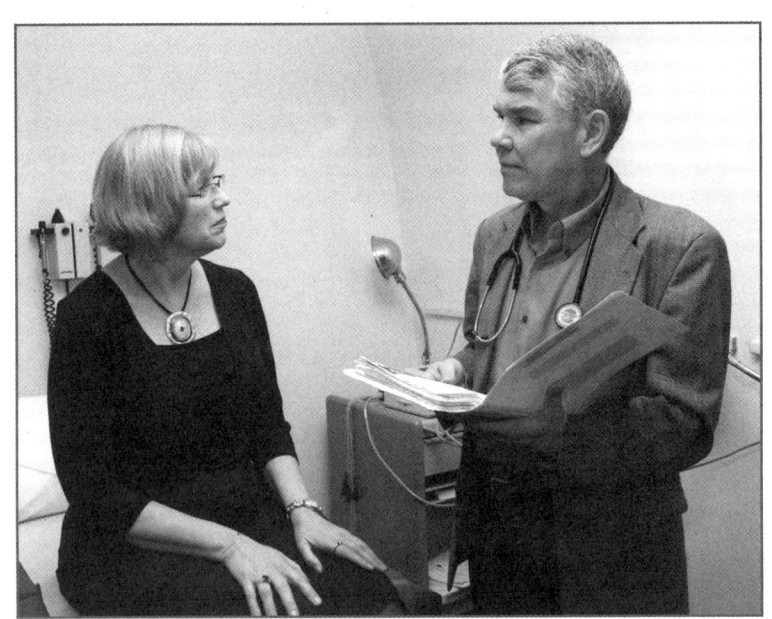

RON HUNNINGHAKE MD
Chief Medical Officer with Center patient.

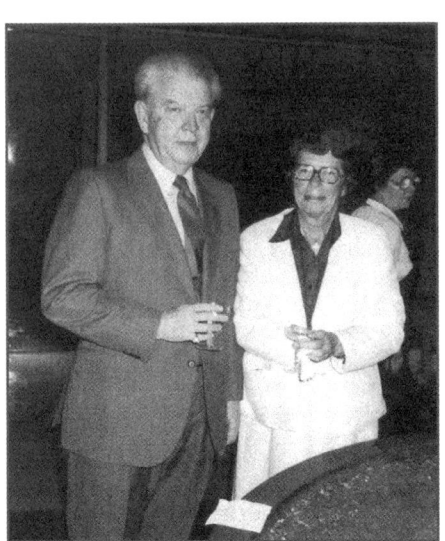

BOB AND MARGE PAGE
Early supporters of Center.

Chapter Five
The Master Facility

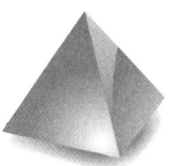

Early in December 1980, after months of study, The Center group decided that the Master Facility would employ primarily Buckminster Fuller's geodesic dome design. It offered the highest degree of cost effectiveness and flexibility to allow expansion.[1] Fundraising for the project began in earnest at the same time. Visits were made to foundations in the Chicago and Detroit areas, particularly Kellogg, McArthur, Stone, and Kresge.[2] But, just as the Koch Foundation had turned down a request to fund "One of a Kind," these proposals also failed to relieve Mrs. Garvey of support for the construction. The Mabee Foundation, however, helped develop the library in the new facility with a $150,000 challenge grant. Perhaps there was not broader support partly because the strong backing of the Garvey family made others feel there was no need.

A campaign began in 1982 to raise local money for the construction. A brochure entitled "Touching the Future" suggested that people "drop your pebble of support into The Center pool of needs and watch with satisfaction as the ripples you generate positively affect so many."[3]

---

1 *Rope*, Dec. 1, 1980.
2 Ibid, Dec. 8, 1980.
3 "Touching the Future," in History Scrapbook #1, CIHF Archives.

Description of the Master Facility and its purposes in various publicity was elaborate:

> We live in a sea of energy. All of life, from tiny subatomic particles to the huge galaxies, can be seen as electro-static and electrodynamic fields. Close examination of life forms, including our own, reveals that the solid state matter of all life exists as waves of energy interacting with one another. It is known that the shape or form of a container affects the nature and quality of the energy force fields within. This is apparent with sound and light and equally so with other portions of the electromagnetic spectrum.

The pyramid, the publicity said, was the ideal structure in which to study the nature of energies too small to feel or measure, and, like the domes, was a solid structure able to withstand any environmental situation. It was so symbolically important that the Founding Fathers had put it on the reverse side of the Great Seal of the United States. People reported that they felt better when inside the pyramid.

The circles were ideal too. The circle was nature's simplest yet most powerful form. The sun was a spherical mass. At its greatest strength the wind took the form of a circle. Tree trunks were circular, the earth's curve was a circle, and so was the action of the ocean's tide. A sphere enclosed the greatest amount of interior space with the least circular area. The form meant 30-50% less heating and cooling than a standard building of the same square footage.[4] As it turned out the operating Center with its heat pumps, earth sheltering, solar technology, and architectural shapes used one half the energy that Kansas Gas and Electric estimated it would.[5] The domes used the strength of numerous triangles to achieve remarkable rigidity with no load-bearing interior walls. As a bonus, they would be a "joy to the senses," blending with

---

[4] Promotional leaflet, n.d. [1982], History Scrapbook #1, ibid.
[5] Interview, Dr. Hugh Riordan with Craig Miner, May 27, 1998.

any setting. Every detail, including the skylights, had a purpose: "The simplicity of its exterior and the sweep of its interior space forms a perfect and harmonious living environment.... People tend to work better, be more productive, study better and suffer less from illness under natural light than artificial full spectrum lighting."[6]

The Center offered to name each of the domes after an individual who provided 51% or more of the funding for any of them. The campaign resulted in Dome #1, the entry to the whole complex, being funded by the Pages and called the Marge Page Dome after the woman who was The Center's first rheumatoid arthritis patient. Dome #2 was called the Mabee Dome, after the major outside foundation contribution. However, the others, for the moment, remained unnamed and entirely funded by Olive Garvey.[7] Eventually, several other domes got funded names, the Betty Marietta Dome, for example, as did a number of areas within them.

In 1981, title to the 90 acres came to The Center, and the model of the Master Facility structures, using "highly evolved architectural forms" to create seven 45-foot and one 60-foot dome, was displayed at the 5th International Conference.[8] In the spring of 1982, Riordan met with an architect in Denver, who he said "fully understands and is well experienced in such important elements as the resonant frequencies of structures, optimum ionization levels, outgassing characteristics of materials, light transmission, solar energy utilization and so much more." He met also with other architects around the country whom he felt were on the leading edge of design. These included some meetings with associates of the Frank Lloyd Wright Foundation in Phoenix and their design for a House of the Future. All these contacts had an effect "upon our capacity to develop a total environment which says to all who come, 'I can be healthier here.'" While the Asian concept of hiring consultants to study the "Chi," or total atmosphere of any building before designing it was commonplace in the late 1990s, in the early 1980s this sort of attention to ambient detail was quite unusual.

---

6 Promotional leaflet, n.d. [1982], History Scrapbook #1, CIHF Archives.
7 *Rope*, April 26, 1982, July 18, 1983.
8 1981 Annual Report in *Rope*, March 11, 1982.

Riordan hoped to stop designing in the spring of 1982 and to move into a new facility by the end of that year.[9] That turned out to be wildly optimistic. However, there was one major and fateful change that spring. In March after a long Wednesday meeting with The Center's architectural firm, PDS, followed by an all-too-common Wednesday evening headache for Dr. Riordan, the thought occurred to him that "what we are wanting to build is a group of imaginative church-like structures rather than a massive concrete and steel building with which the PDS people are more familiar." That realization caused him to call Roe Messner, an area resident who had built 800 churches nationwide. Obviously, Riordan did not have the crystal ball some accused him of consulting and could not know that Messner would later be associated with Jim and Tammy Faye Bakker, that Messner would divert workers from The Center to the Bakker PTL (Praise the Lord) complex, would take bankruptcy, that Jim Bakker would go to prison, and that The Center would end up in the middle of the resultant pile of lawsuits against Messner operations or corporations.

In 1982 it seemed great. Riordan called Messner; Maurice Johnson, the project manager for the Master Facility met with him, and within a week there was the kind of detailed cost analysis and proposal they had been seeking from their former architects for several months. "Subsequent meetings with Roe and his chief architects," Riordan wrote at the time, "made it clear that these were people who understood our mission and who have the expertise, energy, and enthusiasm to make the new master facility become a beautiful reality."[10] Due to what Riordan described as "severe frustrations," the contract with the original architect and builder for The Center was terminated. "It became obvious," he wrote, "that, although they were good people, they were unable to grasp, properly design and cost estimate a building complex that was not to be a standard multi-story concrete and steel building."[11] Messner's firm, Commercial Builders of Kansas, became the contractor for the Master Facility.

---

9 Ibid, March 15, 1982.
10 Letter, Riordan to Olive Garvey, April 1, 1982, Office Files, CIHF Archives.
11 *Rope*, Feb. 18, 1983.

The Master Facility

The push was on. In June, the North Hillside property was contoured, amid regular heavy rains, and a "Skybreaking" was scheduled for July 15, Mrs. Garvey's birthday.[12] On that day the participants released 2,555 tagged balloons, one for each day since The Center had been open, hoping to receive letters back from the finders. They received many back, the furthest one from Illinois.[13] Mrs. Garvey at 89, wrote Marie MacDonald in her *Eagle* column, was a marvel that day as usual. "Although the wind was blowing, not one strand of her beautifully coifed hair was out of place. She was trim as a young girl and her smile just as sweet as it must have been many years ago when it captured the heart of Ray Garvey, her late husband."[14] By the end of July the footings for the first dome were in place.[15] In August, however, it was evident that things were behind schedule, and that there would be no move until the spring of 1983 "or later." 436 N. Bleckley was rented month to month to take the overflow from the other scattered buildings that were then The Center.[16] In October, as the arches and the purloins of the pyramid went up and the structural steel arrived on the rural site, The Center rented an apartment to house the offices of three doctors.[17] By early in 1983, the operation was in four locations in eleven rented apartments and the lab.[18]

The more visible the new and innovative campus became, the more, it seemed, that the attacks on The Center as an institution escalated. There were criticisms from a local Christian Right publication of Marilyn Ferguson, her book *The Aquarian Conspiracy,* and her appearance at The Center's international conference. Ferguson's book, subtitled *Personal and Social Transformation in the 1980s,* was about a transformation of consciousness in the nation that resulted from an explosion of knowledge in all disciplines. And it had a whole chapter on the new

---

12 Ibid, June 14, 1982.
13 Ibid, July 19, 1982.
14 Ibid, Sept., 1982.
15 Ibid, July 26, 1982.
16 Ibid, Aug. 16, 1982.
17 Ibid, Oct. 11, 25, 1982.
18 Ibid, Feb. 18, 1983.

health care, suggesting that "the days of the physician as the sole central figure in the health arena are over."[19]

Ferguson took the word "conspire" in its fundamental Latin sense — "to breathe together," and she saw the future as coming from an accidental but positive paradigm shift. It was only a matter of a "critical number of thinkers" accepting and practicing the new ways.[20] However, the implications that the new mode would change the distribution of power threatened some, and there were some who picked up on the word "conspiracy" to suggest that the left wing was organizing a great attack on traditional values and on the virtues of the establishment. It had started in California (Ferguson was from Los Angeles), but it might well be coming to Kansas, with the lady guru herself as its promoter. After all, she spoke of "humankind embedded in nature;" of the importance of "the myths and metaphors, the prophecy and poetry, of the past;" of the importance of nonconformity and "creative protest;" of the uses of intuition and "transcendental reason;" of "learning as transforming;" of the oneness of life; of "conscious evolution;" of the significance of "networking;" of promoting the "autonomous individual in a decentralized society;" of seeing ourselves as "stewards of all our resources, inner and outer;" of yoga and meditation; of the "transformation of fear;" of the body mind connection; of the importance of relationships; of healing ourselves holistically; of the significance of nutrition to mind and spirit; of trust in oneself, knowing our limits.[21]

This led to attacks from critics. But it was far from a totally negative atmosphere. It was just as Hershey was going to New York to accept the medal for "One of a Kind" that she was responding to the attack.[22] Also then, the *Rope* reported that those "in the know" said no one would come to conferences in Wichita because there were no mountains or ocean, that medicine in Wichita could not get sufficient research funds because

---

19 Marilyn Ferguson, *The Aquarian Conspiracy: Personal and Social Transformation in the 1980s* (Los Angeles: JP. Tarcher, Inc. 1980), 269.
20 Ibid, 19.
21 Ibid, 26, 29, 45, 47, 49, 53, 62, 69, 86-87, 102, 115, 156, 241, 291.
22 Draft of letter from Myrliss Hershey, Oct. 24, 1982, in ibid.

the University was not big enough, it did not have the "necessary" government ties, and researchers would not want to live there. "What those 'in the know' don't know," The Center staff concluded, "is that researchers are asking to come and be part of The Center so that they can work among colleagues who won't laugh at them or degrade them because they perceived non-traditional ways of solving problems."[23] Favorable letters continued to pour in. "If we had more people behind this type of center," one person wrote, "maybe we would have fewer people shooting at presidents, running over law officers and committing fewer acts of violence.... I am only a lay person, but I do know that 800 milligrams of Thorazine a day is enough to frighten the pants off Frankenstein's monster." Another wrote about Mrs. Garvey herself, who had advised President Reagan that his would-be assassin could be helped by The Center, that she was sharper than most 22-year-olds mentally and moved like a much younger person. Many letters were similar to the following:

> In health care as in other areas, it is results that count — whatever works that does no harm. Why in the world are improving one's diet, going for walks, taking a few harmless vitamins and minerals (as opposed to drugs) and even biofeedback labeled as controversial.
>
> In crisis medicine, when one is run over by a truck, certainly drugs and sophisticated methods are life-saving. When one is miserable or dying by inches, less drastic methods work better. In the long run they are cheaper and so improve the utility of life one is happy to live again.[24]

In short, reaction to The Center was complex and varied.

---

23 *Rope*, Dec. 20, 1982.
24 Letters to The Center, n.d. (Sept., 1982), History Scrapbook #1, CIHF Archives. Letter, Olive Garvey to Ronald Reagan, July 22, 1983, Office files, CIHF Archives. The letter was a response to the President's congratulations on Mrs. Garvey's 90th birthday.

In November 1982, lumber for the domes arrived and a crew from Oregon started assembly. A downward trend in the cost of concrete meant that part of the driveway could be concrete rather than the planned asphalt.[25] The Center put an insert in the *Wichita Eagle* about its program and distributed 193,000 brochures in Kansas to counter misinterpretations. *Human News* began its series "The Superb Herb," which was to be long-running and eventually in another publication to educate thousands on that aspect of health.[26] But even the publicity had its glitches. Instead of listing the address of the new facility, one ad gave its longitude and latitude (97 degrees, 17 minutes, 36 seconds, West and 37 degrees, 44 minutes, 22 seconds, North.) The newspaper insert as printed, however, reversed these, making the location appear to be somewhere in outer space over the North Pole. There were a few who found the error quite appropriate.[27]

The year 1983 was a stressful one, mostly due to the construction headaches and delays, combined with hesitation on the part of Garvey about the cost, a staff which had outgrown its facilities, and further charges about CIHF's intentions.

Things started strong enough. The erection of the domes was to start in March and there was a promise they would be in place in a month.[28] That was not far off: the shells of all eight domes were in place by the second week of May, and the pyramid was finished by September.[29] The Center staff offered a course at Friends University entitled "The Psychology and Physiology of Fatigue," which drew nearly 100 students. That was a milestone, which brought together many of the consultants and gave The Center credibility through the university association.[30] The Center put out a proposal to become a resource and development center for world class athletes, documenting the relationship between performance and biochemistry. The program

---

25 *Rope*, Nov. 8, 1982.
26 Ibid, Nov. 15, 1982.
27 Clipping, n.d., History Scrapbook #2, CIHF Archives.
28 *Rope*, Feb. 28, 1983.
29 Ibid, May 9, Sept. 2, 1983.
30 Ibid, Jan. 19, 1983.

had support from local coaches, and The Center hired a second exercise physiologist to help with it.[31] The building plans were expanding, and fundraising calls were being made. Riordan, that "wellspring of ideas and creative plans and programs," as he was called at that time, proposed building a Thaumazein Space in one of the domes that would serve as a state of the art media center.[32] It all seemed suddenly possible. Riordan toured the site in the middle of March, and wrote Mrs. Garvey that he was crying as he composed the note to her. "I don't even know why — except that I am so deeply moved by what you have done for all of us who have been touched by your own caring concern for the well being of people."[33]

It was not long, however, before the headaches again intensified. Riordan personally seemed to suffer more intense insults if not outright attacks than ever before. He was invited, for example, to give the keynote address for the 1984 Kansas Governor's Council on Aging, and accepted. But shortly he received a call from an apologetic lady advising him that the committee had met again and decided that Dr. Riordan was too controversial. A friend of his wrote in response to this rebuff that the Governor's Conference was making "a terrible mistake in not having the genius and talent of Dr. Hugh Riordan at that conference." The CIHF, he thought, "will become one of the most famous and well-known places in Kansas within the next three years and will rival Menningers as a healthcare, health education facility." To shun its founder was "backward thinking."[34] Riordan was reinvited to speak, but refused considering the circumstances.

A second challenge involved his practice on the psychiatric staff at St. Francis Hospital. On December 12, 1983, the psychiatric committee sent Riordan a registered letter that as of December 15 he was no longer to prescribe vitamins and minerals and make dietary adjustments with his hospitalized patients. Riordan contacted medical colleagues

---

31 Ibid, Jan. 31, 1983.
32 Clipping, n.d. [1983], History Scrapbook #1, CIHF Archives.
33 Letter, Riordan to Olive Garvey, March 19, 1983, Office Files, CIHF Archives.
34 *Rope*, Jan. 30, 1984.

and eleven volunteered to testify for him. He then contacted a prominent attorney who knew much of The Center's work and who said he would be glad to help *pro bono*. "I've always wanted to sue them," were his exact words. The attorney wrote a one page letter to the committee, the punch line of which read that if they wanted to go to court and maintain that the standard of psychiatric care in Wichita was to shock, sedate and restrain, Riordan's side would be happy to do so. The order not to change diet disappeared. There was little further opposition there to nutritional therapy.[35]

The episode was certainly distressing to Riordan personally, and perhaps the most upsetting was that his competence in a field where he had practiced for 25 years should be questioned because he was moving beyond it. Laura Benson remembered that, "Dr. Riordan really went through, in my opinion, a lot of pain in those years." The 1983 crisis was one of those times when she wondered how much he could take.[36] As one observer put it, it seemed inevitable that for the moment, "patients who seek nutritional therapy from their physicians will probably be faced with hostile rejection, scorn, amusement, or simply indifference."[37] The same went for physicians who tried to provide such care.

But the biggest headache was money. The projected cost for the Master Facility was running around $4.5 million, operations were expanding, and, to put it briefly, it was not wholly clear where the money was coming from. Late in March, Olive wrote Hugh expressing appreciation that he and his wife, Jan, had been able to visit her in Arizona. "I realize that we did not do what you had hoped, that is, answer specific questions. I also realize the importance these answers have for you because, since I am not immortal, I will not always be the distributor of my charitable funds." Yes, the family believed in him and his mission. "They do want The Center to exist." But they were concerned about two things : 1) that you not expand so fast as to jeopardize qual-

---

35 Interview, Dr. Hugh Riordan with Craig Miner, October 22, 1998.
36 Interview, Laura Benson with Craig Miner, June 10, 1998.
37 A. Hoffer in *Journal of Orthomolecular Psychiatry* in *Rope*, March 5, 1984.

ity or finances, 2) that you not emphasize research to the neglect of clinical services. They understood that The Center's non-profit status with the IRS depended on its research program, but it was the public service part that excited the Garveys the most. Also, she pointed out firmly, she was not made of money. She had invested an "abnormal amount" of her resources in The Center already, was elderly, and could not commit for the long term. "You stated that the clinical services are self-supporting. To have profits you must have production. More production creates more profits. Do you need more doctors to fully utilize the capacity of the laboratory?"[38] That was a business view of things, but there was a lot more to it in Riordan's mind than that. It might be noted, too, that this letter was typed, not hand-written.

Riordan assured her that he would not expand too fast and would keep the clinic and research in balance. But he was projecting ten years into the future, and coming up with a number of $25 million for support. Certainly, some of it would have to come from new sources, but could he depend on "backbone support" from her, at least in the near term? Could she commit to the same level of funding as at present through 1986? "By that time we should have survived the inevitable hostile response which the wonderful Master Facility will bring from my colleagues, and perhaps fundraising would benefit from his writing a book and serving as president of the American Holistic Medical Association.[39]

The family advised finding a fund raiser. Riordan met with Willard Garvey several times, tracked down suggestions, and failed to find one that pleased him.[40] Olive sympathized with the problem. She wrote a fund raising letter herself for The Center, noting that "since most of the world's grief is caused by deranged individuals and chronic illnesses, new knowledge of cause and treatment to alleviate these conditions impresses me as the most productive benefit one could anticipate from use of his money. For this reason, the Olive W. Garvey Center for the Improvement of Human Functioning is my chief object of contribu-

---

38 Letter, Olive Garvey to Riordan, March 23, 1984, Office Files, CIHF Archives.
39 Letter, Riordan to Olive Garvey, April 3, 1983, ibid.
40 Letter, Riordan to Willard Garvey, June 27, 1983, ibid.

tion. But so much needs to be done which my means will not cover. Will you help?"[41] She allowed herself to be interviewed.[42] The Center itself held "ripple lunches" in Wichita to try to generate contributions.[43]

But both she and Riordan knew it was never enough, and that there must be hard choices. She realized, she wrote him, that a progressive program like his

> has no ending. There is constantly an intriguing, promising, compulsive opportunity just ahead. This is as it should be. But also, the stern realities demand that everything has to be paid for. Although opportunities are boundless, finances aren't. There are many things which it is nice to do. We can think of all kinds of reasons why they should be done, but until we can *afford* them financially, they should, in my opinion, be delayed.

It was time for a stricter budget, and a decision on the essentials. "It seems especially easy for institutions depending on contributed capital to persuade themselves they have missions beyond these necessities. I had a battle with Friend's Family Center because it felt it must *give* its services to everyone free of charge. I had to convince them that they were in no financial position to dispense charity. " The same was true of things like free meals and events. "Of course, these gestures are very pleasant. And a certain number of them do provide psychological advantages, promotion and advertisement. But many of them are social cosmetics, and can be eliminated." Here and now, the first priority was to get the Master Facility finished. "If your ram-rod isn't performing, maybe you should replace him." Second was to find new sources of money. Willard thought that the Noble Foundation in Oklahoma was within The Center's grasp and it "has dollars to pennies of our capability."

---

41 Garvey promotional letter, n.d. [1983], in History Scrapbook #2, CIHF Archives.
42 Letter, Olive Garvey to Riordan, Aug. 16, 1983, Office Files, CIHF Archives.
43 *Rope*, Aug. 1, 1983.

She appreciated Riordan's personal sacrifices. "I've made quite a few of those myself. I ran a house and four children on a budget of $100 a month for many years, did considerable manual labor, and denied myself many things. I am no worse for it, and the money I helped save laid the foundation for what others are now spending.... I could be living a 'life of Riley' with airplanes, yachts, and liveried servants if I didn't prefer The Center, you know."[44] He knew.

The two friends were on the platform together again that July 1983, for "Skybreaking" number two. She was 90 that day, would soon receive a Distinguished Services to Mankind Award, and was going strong. She sat in a misty drizzle battling a scratchy throat, but said she could think of no place she would rather be than in front of eight nearly completed geodesic domes and one pyramid, into which she had sunk about $2 million. The Center, with six divisions and a $1 million operating budget, had, she said, "gone far beyond my wildest imaginations. And I feel it's only just starting. I think it will grow and grow.... For a long time I had been thinking that there has to be a better way to treat people who are ill than the way they do it now. And I think this is the way."

Did she see any contradiction between her conservative lifestyle and political views and theories so out of the mainstream as those espoused by The Center, a reporter asked? "No," she answered, "I see no contradiction. I participate in the general health program here and I think it's wonderful. Plus I'm excited about the fact that it's so unique." *Good Morning America* covered the event on ABC national news.[45] The *Wichita Eagle* wrote in an editorial that The Center's "new approach to human health" was a welcome development and "a logical response to the growing knowledge that much of what ails the body is interlinked with one's environment, diet, mental attitude, and a host of other 'non-medical' elements." Olive Garvey, the paper said, was one of Wichita's "grand old ladies." Her "pioneering spirit is helping assure the well-being of future residents of this planet earth." As for the Master

---

44 Letter, Olive Garvey to Riordan, Aug. 16, 1983, Office Files, CIHF Archives.
45 *Wichita Eagle-Beacon*, July 16, 1983, History Scrapbook #2, CIHF Archives.

Facility, there was no question that for Wichita it would be an architectural landmark indeed.[46]

There was tension about the financial challenges, but the friendship between Riordan and Garvey remained as strong as ever. Riordan, she told reporters at the Skybreaking, was "her personal physical guru" and a "medical genius." She added that "We're the Odd Couple, Olive Garvey and Hugh Riordan. He's a miracle worker in my eyes. However, he has not discovered a sure cure for cancer . . . yet."[47] The *Kansas Business News* observed of them that "they make an unlikely team. He's a renegade psychiatrist, the outcast heretic of Wichita's staid medical community. She's one of Wichita's most prominent citizens, a pillar of the community who represents one of the state's largest philanthropic enterprises."

But unlikely or not, the partnership worked, partly because they shared a wise insight. "People are disillusioned with the medical industry," Garvey said. "Escalating costs and the impersonal experimental nature of medicine today has caused more people to look for alternatives in health care." Riordan, she pointed out, was "careful about publicity. He's worried it would appear too sensational. And, it would be." He had, she said, performed real miracles, especially with cancer patients. Riordan himself added: "We try to be on the advancing front. We don't reject standard medicine. We just try to go beyond it. If someone's been helped at The Center, it's either because of or in spite of what we've done. Patients need to discover early on that they're participants in the healing process."[48] That second Skybreaking and attendant publicity were indeed a high point.

In the fall, however, came more reverses. The Garvey Foundation encountered a tax situation which cut its charitable funds by $1 million that year, and it was thought the situation would be permanent. It caused Olive to remind Hugh again of the desirability of finding other funding.[49] The operation had grown enormously. 5,000 people had

---

46 Ibid, July 19, 1983.
47 Ibid, July 16, 1983.
48 *Kansas Business News* (July, 1983) in ibid.
49 Letter, Olive Garvey to Riordan, Sept. 1, 1983, Office Files, CIHF Archives.

been treated since 1975 from 48 states and eight foreign countries, and over 10,000 people had been affected by the conferences. 2,400 had gone through Personal Health Control and the staff had grown from two to 48.[50] Riordan wrote her in September that "much to my surprise the physical reality of the dream appears that it will be even better than the dream itself -- which in my experience is a rare occurrence."[51] He enjoyed, too, the fact that "our new Master Facility is being built near The Center of the nation adequately removed from the unreality of Washington, D.C."[52] But it created strain for him and Garvey knew it. She wrote him that he would make a great president for the Holistic Medicine Association. "On the other hand, it does look like you have a tremendous territory to supervise here, and being of Quaker heritage, I espouse the conviction that example is a powerful influence."[53] He passed up the presidency this time.[54]

That same autumn of 1983, the Garvey Center, a.k.a. "the Kook Factory," was the subject of more attacks from a few people. One woman from Detroit made verbal attacks at a church on September 18, and on a talk show, believing that "our commitment to improving human health is somehow unchristian." Their primary focus was the pyramid, designed for low energy research, but which they equated with Satanic activity. The goal, they said, was to stop The Center from opening. Riordan commented that "although we always anticipate adverse comments from some of our medical colleagues, the attack by these people who profess to be 'true Christians' is a new experience. Since their position is not based upon reason, thoughtful discussion with them is rather impossible." The good news was that as the result of the criticism, The Center had expressions of support from a number of people who had not shown interest before.[55]

A published attack along the same lines appeared on September 30 in a publication called *New Solidarity*. It contained, The Center staff

---

50 Letter, Riordan to Olive Garvey, Sept. 20, 1983, ibid.
51 Ibid, Sept. 25, 1983.
52 Letter, Riordan to "Richard," Sept. 26, 1983, ibid.
53 Letter, Olive Garvey to Riordan, Sept. 23, 1983, ibid.
54 Letter, Riordan to Olive Garvey, Nov. 23, 1983, ibid.
55 *Rope*, Sept. 26, 1983.

said, "a wide variety of preposterous charges about our key people" — so much so that there were talks with attorneys.[56]

The article claimed that threats against a Wichita area National Democratic Policy Committee member had been traced to "an illuminated cult temple and kook factory that just opened for business." It had been linked, the article claimed, to the Lucifer Trust of New York, London, Amsterdam, and Switzerland. It was funded by "a powerful Wichita associate of the Mt. Pelerin Society free-enterprise cult, Olive Garvey," whom the sheet called "the aging and bizarre matriarch of Kansas's most wealthy family." The Center was supposed to be tied to the Nuclear Freeze movement.

The new Center, the article went on, was not for education, but was "a pagan temple built around a huge 'magic pyramid.'" Riordan was a board member of the American Holistic Medical Association which promoted "vitamin and natural medicine kookery." [57]

That sort of thing did not end there. The next spring there was another article in which The Garvey Center was called a "safehouse for cults," and was said to have ties both to the Russian Orthodox Church "which dominates the Soviet KGB" and to the right-wing Nazi International.[58] The Garvey Center was accustomed to criticism, but this was a whole new world of it.

Construction continued, along with the international conferences and invitations to see the actual work being done. 1983 marked the seventh International Conference. 540 health professionals attended, and the organizer, Betty Richards, commented that "new ideas often are branded as weird. And that's OK. We are willing to go out on a limb at both The Center and for our conferences, and we don't let controversy stop us if it's interesting. The controversy is not an issue, but we don't run away from it either." Dr. Callahan was speaking on "Magnetic Monopolies in Holistic Healing," and Dr. William Finley

---

56 Ibid, Nov. 21, 1983.
57 No author listed, "Investigative Leads," in *New Solidarity*, Sept. 30, 1983, in History Scrapbook #2, CIHF Archives.
58 Clips in ibid, Oct. 10, 1983 and April, 1984.

The Master Facility

on "Biofeedback of Evolved Potentials: Implications for Sensory Modification," which concerned his work with paraplegics. In attendance was the medical reporter for the *New York Times*.[59]

Eventually the conferences moved from Century II, both because the Master Facility was available and because a new city policy forced all users of the convention facility to employ a single caterer. The Center's first experience with that caterer was poor, with many complaints about the food. And that could not be allowed to happen. "No matter how wonderful the presentations at a conference," Riordan remarked, "what the people remember is the food."[60]

Those conferences had been a constant educational outreach through the early eighties, and would continue, on a smaller scale, at the Master Facility when it was complete. The 8th conference was to focus primarily on fatigue (the only conference ever devoted to a single subject), and by the 9th one, in 1985, attendance was down to just under 200 because of space limitations.[61] But the expensive rental of the Century II facility was saved, and, in many ways, The Center itself, with its luncheon lectures and its developing newsletter, *Health Hunter*, became a year-round version of the international conferences. The 15th conference was again held at Century II because the new Hyatt Hotel in Wichita provided the food.[62]

Finances remained strained late in 1983. Riordan submitted a funding proposal to the Garvey Foundation which would have, in his opinion, allowed The Center to be self-sufficient by 1986. It was rejected "as being too grandiose." Early in December, he asked for some response about what *would* be possible. With everything he proposed, The Center should not cost more than $5 million: the current building budget was $3 million. That was a lot of money, he admitted, but he marveled that it could be done for what it cost to remodel East High School a few years ago, and for less than the price of a single Lear jet.

---

59 *Wichita Eagle-Beacon*, Sept. 14, 1983, ibid.
60 Interview, Dr. Hugh Riordan with Craig Miner, October 22, 1998.
61 *Rope*, Feb. 21, July 14, 1984, Jan. 28, Sept. 16, 1985.
62 Interview, Dr. Hugh Riordan with Craig Miner, October 22, 1998.

He had no foresight of attacks "from what appears to be the paranoid fringe of some fundamentalist groups," and the Garveys should not be unduly concerned about that.[63]

Olive responded, summarizing a recent Foundation meeting. There were concerns about income. There was enough to complete the building commitment, then a little over $900,000, but she could not "safely promise" to continue the current level of operating subsidy, which was close to $1 million annually. She thought there could be $800,000 in support for 1984, but could not be certain. "I am sure you realize that we would like to be able to furnish all of the things you are planning, but we can't operate on the same principles as those the government uses. We can hope the stock market will be kind." She was taking the thyroid medication Dr. Hugh had recommended, she added, and felt better.[64]

"Thank you," Riordan responded, "for your rapid, if rather disappointing, response.... It seemed appropriate that your letter arrived December 7th since that date has a history of disaster associated with it. We, of course, will deal with the realities of life, and adjust as fully as possible."[65]

As the Master Facility was finished, there continued to be exchanges of this kind. In May 1984, Riordan saw some of the domes lighted from inside for the first time. "I was nearly overwhelmed with a mixture of joy, excitement, awe, appreciation, and trepidation." The trepidation was how this was to be sustained. The Center could add more doctors, but that would not necessarily raise net income, and it could raise its fees, but that would contradict Olive's desire of making the place affordable for as many as possible. But the Foundation had cut its funding for 1984 by $400,000 and it was causing a pinch. "If there is to be a severe lessening of support before we are able to sustain ourselves, why have you helped us to go this far -- to be born after a nine-year gestation. I very much need to know if our goal is to sell off the Master Facility and work in isolation serving a very few or if our

---

63 Riordan to Olive Garvey, Dec. 4, 1983, Office Files, CIHF Archives.
64 Olive Garvey to Riordan, Dec. 6, 1983, ibid.
65 Riordan to Olive Garvey, Dec. 8, 1983, ibid.

goal is to be in the year 2000 the most outstanding health-medical facility in the world?"[66]

He understood he was pushing. "Perhaps by now you are saying, 'Is this man crazy?' 'He seems to be asking for more money after I have done so much.' Probably I am a little crazy — about the Olive W. Garvey Center…what we have done and what we can do." He had had a decrease of 50% in personal income, and given up his $1,000 a day consulting fee. He therefore took the success of The Center very personally.[67]

Olive was sympathetic, but firm. In August 1984, shortly after The Center had seen its first patient at the Master Facility, she wrote:

> I will have to answer again that one does not get milk out of a turnip. We may be able to help a little more in completing necessary details. But this is all we can promise. There has to be a practical, precise plan made and followed.
>
> You have invested nine years. I have invested not much less than that many million dollars. We have both laid our reputations on the line. We are equally anxious that our investment be sound and that it will accomplish its advertised purpose.
>
> It seems to me that to accomplish that end it is necessary to tie up all the threads of the enterprise at this point…. I know how many wonderful things there are out there which will add to the program in innumerable ways. I know it is like the chicken and egg: they are desirable and they will bring in incomes. But I think they must be kept in abeyance until the foundation is firm and paid for….

---

66 Ibid, May 8, 1984.
67 Ibid, Aug. 13, 1984. Interview, Dr. Hugh Riordan with Craig Miner, October 22, 1998.

Probably your greatest problem is that you are too capable in too many lines. You are undoubtedly a better physician, and a better money-raiser and publicist than anybody you can hire. It is extremely annoying and requires superhuman patience to let somebody else do what you can do better. Almost every really capable person has this problem to put up with.

But, after all, you, yes, even you, are mortal. You may get along on four hours sleep a night, but I've seen you looking mighty weary, and you won't always be 52….

The primary need is money, and money has to be cared for and managed. [68]

That letter, Riordan responded, was, as usual "caring, perceptive, and candid." He wanted his response to be the same. His financial situation was less strong than when he was in private practice. He understood the foundation was required by law to give away money and such giving did not necessarily reflect a personal monetary commitment from those involved. Yet, The Center needed administration. "We have looked to our own ranks and now have two co-administrators." These were Dr. Myrliss Hershey for human resources and Laura Benson for fiscal matters. The Center was programmed to decrease its request from the Foundation until it was self-supporting in 1987. "I realize that my perfectionist tendencies can lead to disappointments in terms of staff performance." But he wanted highly effective people so that he could be a physician and the international spokesman. "I also am fully aware of my mortality particularly as I attend the ever more frequent funerals of my contemporaries. Although I have no apparent physical complaints or plans for dying soon, weariness does periodically creep into my being especially when it is necessary to cut staff due to less than sufficient funds as was the case this year. I am both flattered and slightly wearied by the perception that my commitment to The Center is so strong that only death could take me from it."

---

68 Olive Garvey to Riordan, Aug. 17, 1984, ibid.

The Master Facility

He outlined the financial details. There was $390,000 in the bank, $330,000 in construction-related bills, $100,000 payable from the sale of the lab building on Douglas, service income of $50,000 a month, and expenses of $110,000 to $120,000 a month. It was indeed a chicken and egg situation. Without $500,000 in cash on hand, other foundations would be less likely to support The Center. At present there was real strain.[69]

There was some movement. The Foundation sent an extra $100,000, and it promised to keep the support level in 1985. But, Olive wrote, "you know if we give capital we soon have no income for next year."[70] In 1983, the CIHF had expended $1,704,361.99 on operations, of which $1,200,000 came from Garvey sources. In addition $790,029.86 was spent that year on the Master Facility, all of it coming from Garvey. There were more $1,000 contributions than ever. Non-Garvey contributions were up 14% from the year before. The Society had 600 members. Sales of books and tapes were up. But it was obvious that the Development Division "was less than cost effective." It was also obvious that the prospect that the Garvey support would be reduced by 1/3 (or over $400,000) in 1984 was "a significant blow."[71]

None of that was public. Amid the night ruminations and the belt-tightening, a remarkable facility was completed. The *Wichitan* magazine in November 1983, called it a "Holistic Holidome." When The Center was founded in 1975, the reporter recalled, "some of its ideas were thought to be far out California-trendy theories," but in 1983 Wesley Hospital had a wellness center, and Koch Industries, and several local aircraft companies sponsored wellness programs. So it did not look so far out anymore. There was a 60 foot diameter dome, surrounded by seven 45 foot ones, all connected by underground tunnels. The pyramid was 60 x 60 feet at the base and 39 feet high, the entire complex comprising about 50,000 square feet. The Garvey Founda-

---

69 Riordan to Clifford Allison, Oct. 2, 1984, ibid.
70 Riordan to "People," Oct. 13, 1984, Olive Garvey to Riordan, Nov. 13, 1984, ibid.
71 Annual Report, 1983, in *Rope*, Feb. 21, 1984.

tion had contributed $3 million for the construction. "Although The Center is biochemically oriented," Riordan told the magazine, "we strongly believe in the benefits of the whole person approach with each patient. Consideration of the whole person includes analysis of physical, nutritional, environmental, emotional and lifestyle values as well as the recognition of each person being an active and responsible participant in the healing process rather than a passive victim of a disorder or a passive recipient of treatment."[72]

Many asked what was "The Improvement of Human Functioning?" As tours of The Center began, a sheet was available to answer that. The Center specialized, it said, in "complicated chronic illness" which was not helped by standard diagnosis and treatment, as judged by the patient. Such patients usually exhibited a "highly individual disordering of several biochemical parameters…. Taken separately, any of these metabolic abnormalities would probably not exhibit sufficient causative power to shape the patient's symptom/disease complex. Taken together, their cumulative effect disrupts cellular function in a global manner, touching multiple organ systems and manifesting as complex chronic illness." The Center could "improve the functioning" of such people and their quality of life.[73] It cost $45 for admission, $75 for a first visit, and then costs depended on the malady. "We don't really do anything in the way of patient care that's really off the wall," Riordan said. The newspaper publicity surrounding the completion of the campus collected the comments of both supporters and detractors on that philosophy. There were plenty of both. Patients were ready with testimonials. Marge Page said that her Center regimen meant "I get up eager each morning and am never exhausted by evening. The energy level is the amazing result that everyone I know in this program has experienced. Needless to say, I am a complete convert to Dr. Riordan's approach to medicine." Louise Greiner, from southwest Kansas, was another. She had been hospitalized 24 times in the past two years with heart problems until The Center found she was sensitive to a dozen

---

72 *Wichitan* (Nov., 1983), 38-39 in History Scrapbook #2, CIHF Archives.
73 Internal draft n.d. [1984] in ibid.

foods. Her heart returned to a regular beat when she avoided these foods, she was off medication and only returned once every six months for a check. Riordan himself said he was able to overcome his afternoon fatigue by switching from black to red pepper on his lunch salads, and was able to stop wearing glasses for astigmatism through using a correct diet. Olive Garvey said her arthritis stopped hurting after she gave up white potatoes. Satisfied patients ranged from a US ambassador to a Dallas Cowboys cheerleader.

Riordan, however, stated only the obvious in saying, "I don't think there's been any shortage of critics." Cytotoxic testing was much in dispute, and Wichita physicians questioned The Center's use of it to find food sensitivities. In fact the whole idea that food sensitivity was important to any but a few people was doubted. There was no experimental evidence, local doctors said, that diet affects health in the dramatic ways described: there were only individual patient stories --the zeal of converts. Many physicians said that large doses of vitamins and minerals might be dangerous. Others said that they were just unnecessary, creating "expensive urine." The Director of the Sedgwick County Medical Society said he knew of no organized opposition to the Garvey Center by doctors or hospitals, but there was skepticism. Most doctors, he said, viewed it as experimental, and patients should see their family doctor before taking treatment there. [74]

Yet, it was done. There was a third Skybreaking on Olive's 91st birthday, July 15, 1984. To mirror the frustrations of the other such events, the Master Facility was still not quite ready. But it was close this time. There were 3,300 balloons. And, amid the pressures and pains, it still seemed worth it.[75]

"I'm sure," said Mrs. Garvey, that "the past two years have furnished a grueling demonstration of the ability to deal with frustration and aggravation caused by the endless changes and delays which have accompanied this erection of an innovative structure which planners and inspectors seem not able to comprehend. The fact that the staff

---

74 *Wichita Eagle-Beacon*, July 14, 1984, ibid.
75 Ibid.

is still in good health and philosophical good humor, proves that they have a workable method for dealing with that celebrated stress …. I am persuaded that the potential for this institution is limitless: it has the concept, it has the interest of the top-level physicians and researchers, it has the plant for expansion."

It had, as well "a high record of success in the improvement of daily well-being for hundreds of people and cases of phenomenal cures." And it had a dream to "become not only a landmark for mid-America, but a benchmark for the human race."

Hugh Riordan also spoke, noting that all were there that hot July day because Roger Williams first stimulated Olive Garvey's thinking about nutrition. They were there because of Fowler Poling, MD who had told Riordan that they could keep people out of the state hospital by giving them vitamin B. They were there because of people like Carl Pfeiffer. They were there because there were more and more people who thought it was absurd that so many Americans lived so much of their lives in poor health, and, what was more, hardly knew what they were missing. The prayer for the occasion was given by Dr. Jon Sward: "Enable us to hear nature's music, to break out dancing, coming alive, taking risks, choosing alternatives, and being the life you've created us to be."[76]

Dr. Riordan told a reporter that day that, "we're still considered in a quack area by a lot of people. Within 10 years we could be doing Nobel (prize) quality work." Olive Garvey said she had "just about sunk everything I've got into it." She ignored statements that it was a rich woman's folly. "I think there's skepticism in everything." The local paper agreed that it was amazing, but wasn't sure it was appropriate. "In an alfalfa field north of Wichita, the eight gleaming white geodesic domes look as out of place as Eskimo igloos. Then there's the pyramid."[77]

There was an Associated Press story, not only about the buildings, but about the program. Riordan told that reporter that, "when you're functioning optimally, it's like a reservoir dam that's not only full but

---

76 Text of July, 1984 Skybreaking, in History Scrapbook #1, CIHF Archives.
77 *Wichita Eagle-Beacon,* July 14, 1984, History Scrapbook #2, CIHF Archives.

slopping over just a little." He said the best co-learners were cattlemen who were used to supplementing their livestock's feed with vitamins and minerals. Robert Reeve, a food and nutrition professor at Kansas State University, was caustic about that, commenting that "they are certainly enriching the sewer system of the city of Wichita." To that kind of comment the staff just responded that they were "victims of an emotional debate that is decades behind the current research." Said Marv Dirks: "We're hard-core scientific about measuring where people stand [biochemically] and seeing what they need."[78]

After some structural fixes, and some fine adjustments, the CIHF moved into its Master Facility late in August 1984.[79] The buildings continued for some time to get publicity. Rising like "a strange breed of mushroom," went one article, it looked like a movie set for a George Lucas production. And there were still brickbats thrown about what went on there. Would the claims of cures stand up under close scrutiny, doctors asked, or did these people suffer from psychosomatic ailments, see the Garvey Center as the last resource, and will themselves back to health?[80]

Patiently, Riordan continued to respond. "There is a prevailing assumption," he said,

> that we only get sick because we are attacked by 'invaders.' For this reason, most research and treatment is directed at learning how to destroy the invaders once they have caused illness and disease. At The Center, we find the fact of great significance that many people do not become sick even though the same invaders attack them. We believe those who are less prone to becoming ill have more adequate reserves and therefore are healthier. Our approach recognizes that the human mind and body are magnificent instruments designed

---

78 *Salina Journal,* July 15, 1984, ibid.
79 *Rope,* Jan. 16, Aug. 20, 1984.
80 Clip in *Rope,* from *Wichita Pizzaz,* October, 1984.

to perform well without disease and disability, provided their needs for adequate to optimal functioning are recognized and met. Disease and disability are not viewed as inevitable results from living in a hostile environment. Rather they are viewed as the result of a prolonged period of depleted reserves. When people who once viewed themselves as helpless victims under attack begin to see themselves as "builders of their reserve," their non-helpful fears and anxieties change to feelings of hope and optimism. That is why our treatment programs, research and educational efforts are geared toward helping people discover their own unique requirements and developing their reserves.[81]

That was the reason for the whole thing — pyramid, domes, tunnels, and all.

Dr. Riordan wrote in his annual report to supporters that the year 1984 could best be described by words such as "expectation, delay, fulfillment, transition, anguish, frustration, creative problem solving, combining skills, stretching capacities, and above all reality."[82] In short it was a typical year of ups and downs for The Center, just a bit more intense. When Riordan gave a talk at the American Holistic Medicine Association convention that year called "Challenges Facing the Holistic Physician," he knew whereof he spoke.[83] But there was great hope, too. Mrs. Garvey had written, shortly after she was given the Kansan of the Year Award for 1984, that "if America is to survive, it will have to take its program from Kansas and the Mississippi Valley."[84] That sounded like the pre-Dust Bowl days in Kansas when it was seen as a vanguard and a beacon, not a backwater.

---

81 Vickie Griffith Hawver in *Topeka Capital-Journal*, Oct. 14, 1984, in History Scrapbook #2, CIHF Archives.
82 Annual Report, 1984, in *Rope*, March 4, 1985.
83 Flyer for AHMA meeting, May, 1984, in History Scrapbook #2, CIHF Archives.
84 *Wichita Eagle-Beacon*, January 28, 1984, ibid.

And, certainly, the Master Facility was a great and irreplaceable asset for The Center, both in function and in visibility and symbolism. The *Rope* crowed late in 1984 that "together, without a single dime of government tax money and its attendant bureaucratic intervention and control, without even a single strand of string attached to or from any special interest group, without a single penny owed on our magnificent Master Facility in its present state of completion, we have been able to see the Olive W. Garvey Center for the Improvement of Human Functioning, Inc., become a reality."[85] The Pyradomes, as they were sometimes called, were certainly "unlike any other place on earth."[86]

---

85 *Rope*, Dec. 24, 1984.
86 Brochure "Tour the Pyradomes," n.d., History Scrapbook #1, CIHF Archives.

Chapter Six
Health Hunters

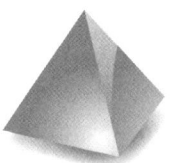

The new physical facility was, for a time, a monumental distraction. The staff got out the buckets every time it rained and watched attorneys struggle.

Roe Messner had been a great hope in the beginning. After two years of facilities planning meetings with the former architects, and all the Wednesday headaches with no solid beginning, Messner had told Riordan that, yes, he could build a pyramid (the former firm was having trouble with this) as well as the domes, and, yes, he could get going right away, using his church-building experience in all climates and topographies to solve the problems.[1]

There were some problems during the construction. There were cracks in the concrete, especially near the skylights, requiring the entire tunnel structure to be resealed. One week vandals did considerable damage to one of the domes, operating the sheet rock crew's electric platform to push one of the domes off its foundation. Extra waterproof membrane, not in the original plan, was put over all the tunnel tops.[2] But it seemed the planning was ultra-careful. The Center staff was especially aware of

---

[1] Interview Dr. Hugh Riordan with Craig Miner, Sept. 15, 1998.
[2] *Rope*, Jan. 16, 1984.

the effect of "environmental factors on our sense of well-being." The plan allowed a two-week period, for instance, between the carpet laying and moving in to allow the glue used to outgas.[3] There were soon leaks — leaks everywhere it seemed. Kansas was a relatively dry place, but spring rains in Wichita could be far too torrential to allow any gaps.

The first attempt at a fix was to apply extra waterproofing on the lower level walls to try to plug over 40 identified leaks. That was done in February 1985 and failed to solve the problem completely.[4] To make things worse, the original waterproofing contractor placed a lien on the property for non-payment of $2,000 of the $56,000 charge for waterproofing that did not waterproof. The attitude was that they were not responsible, a stance that seemed bizarre to The Center staff and totally alien to its philosophy. Lawsuits were threatened. The stress was high because The Center had tried hard to stick to its construction budget and keep the facility debt free. There were slight overruns due to city regulation compliance and changes in the paving, but these had been covered by the Garvey and Page families. Litigation costs and extensive extra waterproofing were another matter. That would certainly quash plans for attracting a group of investors to purchase wind generators for the master facility, as had been hoped. One consolation was that since, for the moment, the development office remained unfilled, the Garvey Center had "the highest ratio of funds generated to fund-raising expenses of any organization known to exist."[5]

"Teething" problems continued to plague the new facility. An innovation, for instance, had been a gate system at the entrance activated by pressure. The idea was that at night barriers would rise in the middle of the driveway which would lower for people coming out of The Center, but would not let people in after a certain hour. The sensors for these, however, continuously malfunctioned, and they eventually had to be replaced with standard gates.[6] Cutting the alfalfa which still

---

3 Ibid, April 30, 1984
4 Ibid, Feb. 11, 1985.
5 Ibid, March 4, 1985.
6 Ibid, July 1, 1985.

grew on the acreage provided some income or material for use, but there was some incompatibility between operating a farm and running a health center.[7] In August 1985, lightning hit one of the domes and did $20,000 worth of damage to computers and telephones.[8]

The leak difficulty, however, was the worst, and it extended for a long time. In January 1987, The Center filed suit in Sedgwick County District Court against Commercial Builders, who blamed subcontractors and defective materials for the continuing problems. The Center argued it was inadequate design and negligent construction. Attorneys for subcontractors Global Coating and Midwest Drywall promised that their clients would try to remedy part of the problems, but that action was slow and inadequate ("the two main subcontractors began blaming each other rather than completing the work") and the lawsuit caused a delay in plans to have the entire outer surface recoated and waterproofed. Every time it rained the drill was to go around collecting evidence for the litigation. In the spring of 1987 discovery conferences were held and a consulting engineer from Kansas State University was retained. He concluded that there were serious design flaws as well as construction defects, and that the reinforcement material in the concrete was shorted. That would constitute fraud on the part of Commercial Builders. In November Commercial Builders offered to settle by giving The Center $45,000 cash and assigning it any rights it had against their insurance company. That was rejected.[9]

As litigation dragged on something had to be done. Therefore, in the summer of 1988, all the domes were recoated with an inch or more of waterproof urethane. The final two coats were white, but the undercoats were yellow and black, making for some dramatic photographs.[10] This process disrupted the business of The Center considerably (it had to close for two weeks) but fixed most of the aboveground leaks.[11]

---

7 Ibid, July 15, 1985.
8 Ibid, Aug. 5, 1985.
9 Ibid, Feb. 25, 1988.
10 Ibid, Aug. 15, 1988.
11 Annual Report 1988 in *Rope*.

Finally, in October 1989, the civil suit against the contractor began.[12] It ran 16 days, leading Riordan to comment that it was the longest period of time he had sat in such a way since he learned to walk. The case went to the jury in November, and by a vote of 11-1 the jury awarded The Center damages of $918,000. Midwest Drywall was found liable for $16,500 of the damages. The problem was collecting. Commercial Builders resisted the judgment. Meanwhile The Center was paying interest on a $186,000 loan, the first debt it had ever had, for the 1988 recoating of the domes. In addition the entire staff took a 10% reduction in pay for two months to help finance the recoating. It was hard to imagine most medical facility staffs being willing to do that and was a tribute to the relationships that had been established. Even were the entire settlement collected, it would not be enough to make the needed repairs, but it was a sort of moral victory at least.[13]

The agony on that front went on and on. In January 1990, The Center inquired why it had not been paid when Messner's company, Commercial Builders, still had equipment, and was near completing a $28,000,000 14,000 seat church in Tennessee. True, with the Bakker scandal, Messner had quite enough trouble, and The Center denied that it was trying to put him out of business. But it seemed fair for it to have an early claim on the firm's income.[14] The Center's attorneys claimed that Messner was transferring money out of Commercial Builders into other companies.[15]

In March 1990 the "financially embattled" Messner sought bankruptcy protection. His companies had debts over $11 million and "disputed debts" of an additional $21 million. The September previous, Commercial Builders of Kansas, Messner's design and construction company, had filed for reorganization. Bakker was in jail and his Heritage USA Christian retreat in South Carolina was bankrupt

---

12 *Rope*, Oct. 16, 1989.
13 Ibid, Nov. 13, 1989. *Wichita Eagle*, Dec. 13, 1989, History Scrapbook #3, CIHF Archives. Interview, Dr. Hugh Riordan with Craig Miner, October 22, 1998.
14 *Wichita Business Journal*, Jan. 29, 1990, History Scrapbook #3, CIHF Archives.
15 Interview, Dr. Hugh Riordan with Craig Miner, October 22, 1998.

and unable to pay Commercial Builders, which was its prime contractor. Bakker's organization, Praise the Lord, sometimes better known as "Pass the Loot" by those who knew it best, owed Messner $15 million. Messner was also in trouble on the elaborate Terradyne Country Club development at his home town of Andover, Kansas. The Central Bank of Walnut Creek, California, in February 1990, filed an $8.6 million foreclosure action involving that project. Messner and his wife had defaulted on personal guarantees but were allowed to continue to operate under Chapter 11 bankruptcy reorganization. At the time of the Chapter 11 filing, the Garvey Center award was Commercial Builders' largest liability, but a $750 million PTL-related lawsuit, accusing Bakker and others in his organization of diverting millions to their own purposes, had named Messner as a defendant.[16]

That spring of 1990 there was an auction scheduled of 3,000 items seized from Commercial Builders of Kansas, worth an estimated $200,000. The sale of that equipment was to satisfy at least part of the debt owed The Center under the court judgment. However, the federal bankruptcy judge stopped the auction after the bankruptcy filing.[17] In October Commercial Builders filed Chapter 7 bankruptcy, meaning that it was ceasing operations completely, and that its creditors would have to get in line to collect from any remaining assets.[18] The Center collected only minimal sums.

Of course there were brighter spots. In March 1985 The Center held its first formal training for volunteers: there were eight people in that class.[19] A Center volunteer support group was formed called Delta Sigma Gamma, which stands for "Doing Something Good." Volunteers have been an integral part of The Center, especially in the new building, and they have had a variety of assignments, certainly not limited to the kind of help for which people are easily "trained" and readily interchangeable. Instead of fitting the volunteers into a pre-ordained

---

16 *Wichita Eagle,* March 3, 1990, ibid.
17 Ibid, Feb. 2, March 9, 1990.
18 *Rope,* Oct. 15, 1990.
19 Ibid, March 11, 1985.

job, the staff started with the person and adjusted the program to fit his or her strengths. They did everything from working with Dr. Riordan, working with nurses and *pro tem*, and helping with the computer and library. They also assisted in the kitchen, with the mailings, and in financial support. These volunteers were often former patients who were grateful and were giving back. In 1999 volunteerism averaged about 6,000 hours a year from 22 regular volunteers and others who gave time for big special events. A number of volunteers made the transition to paid staff.[20]

The Center started a garden at its new facility and planned that summer to sell vegetables and herbs grown organically. There were plans to grow nutrition-rich experimental plants in a solar greenhouse one day.[21] Project ATTUNE, a two-week camp, started in June in cooperation with Wichita State University. 35 high potential, low achievement children, ages 9-17, spent some time at The Center gaining insight on improving their performance and perhaps becoming educated as future supporters of alternative medicine. There was follow up during the school year.[22] A nutritionally-sound restaurant, *The Taste of Health*, started with Nanda Langston in charge.[23] It served lunch Monday-Friday for $4, considerably below cost. The day the *Wichita Eagle* food reviewer ate at The Center, the menu included steamed carrots, freshly baked bread, fruit cup, skinless chicken teriyaki, apple honey custard pie and herbal iced tea.[24] Then, as ever after, The Center's restaurant provided healthful food that was tasty and sold at a reasonable price. It seemed a perfect way to transition local people away from meals that were creating customers for the cardiac specialists. The only problem was that as a non-profit, The Center could not advertise the restaurant or even put up a sign at the entrance about it. Therefore it remained to some degree a delicious secret of The Center's patrons and supporters. But The Center itself was not

---

20 Interview, Laura Benson and Marilyn Landreth, Aug. 19, 1999.
21 *Rope*, April 8, 1985.
22 Ibid, June 17, July 8, 1985.
23 Ibid, July 15, 1985.
24 *Wichita Eagle Beacon* , Nov. 29, 1985, History Scrapbook #2, CIHF Archives.

so much a secret as before. "Come walk, crawl or run with Dr. Hugh," went a flyer in 1985 (Bob Page with his wry sense of humor had, as a condition of a gift for the trail insisted on a sign forbidding jogging). "Come move your body where birds share their songs, frogs croak, deer sometimes appear and the doctors share their thoughts. Come move your body around — JUST FOR THE HEALTH OF IT."[25]

Important to maintaining all that was fundraising. In March, Riordan reported to Olive Garvey that "at long last a person has come along who fulfills the qualifications I have been looking for in a Director of Development." That person was Richard Lewis.[26] Lewis, a native of El Dorado, Kansas, was 50 years old, had a degree in English, background in engineering and math, job experience ranging from construction to aviation, and a wife who was a dean at Wichita State University.[27]

Like many Center employees, his background was not specific to the cause: he was older, was a manager at a steel company, and had no particular experience either in health care or in fund raising work. His resume was sent to Riordan by a friend and would probably not have been considered by most parallel organizations. But Riordan saw qualities in the man, particularly after meeting him, and was willing to back his intuition with opportunity. Lewis had been in the first Personal Health Control group, believed in the program, and was articulate. It was said, too, that he understood long hours and had "an ability to tolerate frustration."[28] In addition, Riordan observed, "he has sufficient fortitude and self confidence to work easily with me without being intimidated; he has attained sufficient maturity to maintain a resilient perspective in the face of inevitable rejection experienced by those asking for money, and every member of our staff who has met him likes him and looks forward to his being with us." To Riordan the fact that he had never been a fund raiser before was the best part. He had no baggage about how the job should be done and no feeling that it couldn't be done.[29]

---

25 Flyer, n.d. [1985], History Scrapbook #2, CIHF Archives.
26 Letter, Riordan to Olive Garvey, March 16, 1985, Office Files, CIHF Archives.
27 Staff Profiles, Mabee Library, CIHF.
28 *Rope*, April 1, 1985.
29 Letter, Riordan to Olive Garvey, March 16, 1984, Office Files, CIHF Archives.

Lewis was eating a bad diet when he started at The Center. "I wasn't heavy," he recalled, "but I loved food. I loved heavy food, rich cooking, lots of fats." He phased out of that slowly but surely, and his health improved. After a time eating fat made him feel that his mouth was coated as though he had been drinking a cup of lard. The same was true of eating lower amounts of salt. A regular restaurant meal would then make one feel that "you're eating brine soup." They were small changes perhaps, but they were real and Lewis, like so many other employees changed his own views about The Center. "Most people had a strange idea about what The Center was," Lewis noted in 1998. "They still do. When you kind of keep a low profile, myth rushes in to fill the void." The public impression often was that "we were just an exclusive club that did strange things."

Lewis ended up doing many jobs besides development. His role as a tour guide, for instance, began one day when Riordan overheard him talking to some friends about The Center and decided he was very good at it.[30] But development was his start, and it was a necessary focus for the organization in its post construction era. Olive Garvey made a special gift of $100,000 to start the development program under Lewis. She noted in her letter confirming this that he would be expected in the future to support his own work, and that, incidentally, she had heard that Riordan had cured people with "imbalance." That and chronic bronchitis were two of her long-term health problems she had given up on. As always the funding, the friendship, and the professional work were all mixed up in the making of the institution.[31]

Garvey and Riordan took the occasion of the hiring of Lewis to negotiate again about the kind of gap outside funding would be expected to fill. Riordan wrote her in September that he would like $800,000 from her in 1986, $600,000 in 1987, $400,000 in 1988, $200,000 in 1989, and that he would have The Center fully self-supporting in 1990.[32] She responded with the usual caution that she did not make fund-

---

30 Interview, Richard Lewis with Craig Miner, June 3, 1998.
31 Letter, Olive Garvey to Riordan, March 26, 1985, ibid.
32 Letter, Riordan to Olive Garvey, Sept. 22, 1985, ibid.

ing promises beyond one year, but that the 1986 amount would be fine and "the remainder of your requests look reasonable, and barring some unforeseen circumstances happening to either The Center, or to Garvey Foundation, we think you will be justified in depending on the remainder of your requests being granted."[33] That represented comparative certainty for planning, and a definite challenge in fundraising. And it had always been true, and no doubt would continue to be true, that Olive would fund one of Hugh's special ideas now and then, just out of curiosity to see how it would work and whether she could help start something that could be important to many far into the future.

Lewis hosted some events that made a little money and attracted potential large givers to The Center. In June 1985, for example, there was a gala evening for research that raised $15,000 with an expense of $6,000.[34] The goal was to raise $20 million in ten years for research, and the vision was to have Nobel quality work done at The Center.[35]

As had always been the case, there were regular approaches to foundations, with the regular result that the work of the Garvey Center was too different from the standard. In the fall of 1986, for instance, the Wesley Foundation rejected a request from The Center for a matching grant of $4,500 to conduct nutritional studies on individuals with Down's Syndrome.[36] Again in 1988 it rejected a Center request for joint research with Wichita State University on the links between cancer and the lack of specific amino acids and trace minerals.[37] James Landsdowne of the Foundation personally supported Riordan and thought that the Foundation should back some of its work. But there was objection among the medical staff.[38]

Mostly, therefore, The Center looked to individual, private donors to fund its research. In 1985, for instance, there was a proposed chelation

---

33 Letter, Olive Garvey to Riordan, Sept. 24, 1985, ibid.
34 *Rope*, July 15, 1985.
35 *Wichita Eagle Beacon*, June 19 1985, History Scrapbook #2, CIHF Archives.
36 *Rope*, Sept. 29, 1986.
37 Ibid., Jan. 18, 1988.
38 Interview, James Landsdowne with Craig Miner, Spring, 1998.

study, which would require $100,000.[39] Called, "Get the Lead Out," it was occasioned by recent studies that showed the average American had 500 times the lead in the body as ancestors of two generations ago.[40] The problem for The Center was, as Riordan later put it, that chelation "was interfering with the cottage industry of cardiovascular surgery."[41]

Late in 1984 The Center got word that the Kansas Board of Healing Arts was meeting to consider making intravenous chelation illegal in the state. And it was "the pressure being brought to bear" that occasioned the research project, designed to educate the pubic and the legislators as well as advance science. A doctor backing the study called the move against chelation a "Galileo effect." Galileo was brought before the Inquisition not because of his astronomical theories so much as because he chose to go directly to the public with them before the powers of the Church could decide on a party line in response. "Chelation therapy is a threat to a $5 billion per year industry," it was noted. "One must expect some politically and economically motivated attempts at reprisal." But there was anger that chelation was called "dangerous." It had been used on over 300,000 patients with not more than 15 whose deaths could be even remotely related to chelation, and in every case this was because it was administered improperly. Even accepting that all these deaths were truly from chelation, it was still 200 times safer than bypass surgery. Wrote another doctor in a supporting letter for The Center's intervention with the state Board of Healing Arts: "Those who stress surgical over non-surgical therapies tend to ignore the neurological, molecular, cellular, enzymatic, and hormonal factors in occlusive arterial disease. Arteries are dynamic, muscular structures which expand and contract in response to varied stimuli." Dr. Riordan sent all these letters to the state board with the comment in his cover letter that "it is my strong hope that the rumor mill is inaccurate and that you are not even considering such a blatant intrusion upon the freedom of physicians in Kansas to

---

39 *Rope.*, Sept. 9, 1985.
40 News Release, Nov. 11, 1985 in *Rope*.
41 Interview, Dr. Hugh Riordan with Craig Miner, June 3, 1998.

provide what in their judgment and experience is effective treatment."[42] The Center received $10,000 from the Amen Trust right away for the chelation study and $10,000 from the Garvey Foundation.[43]

Related was the Pepper bill of early 1985. Again the threat was turned into a public relations opportunity for The Center, and it followed up with attempts at financial development. It was a well-known fact that people often gave money in response to a perceived threat to something they valued more readily than they did simply to advance the fortunes of an institution they considered secure.

The Pepper bill, sponsored by Claude Pepper, the congressional champion of the elderly, was to establish a strike force on health quackery. This team was to eradicate "drugs, medical devices, and medical treatment procedures which are *known* to be fake or whose safety and effectiveness are not proven." That much seemed admirable, but the language of the bill was very broad. Who would determine what was safe? Aspirin was reported to cause 10,000 deaths a year. "Science is a constantly evolving field," wrote one critic of the Pepper bill. "Today's facts often become tomorrow's quackery. Bleeding and purging were the *rule* in George Washington's time."[44] The Center worried that the Pepper task force might take aim at a number of their procedures, including the use of large doses of vitamins, something that was under almost constant attack in the press. Should the Pepper bill pass, the word internally at The Center was, it would "virtually eliminate our capacity to function as we believe."[45] There was a sigh of relief on North Hillside when the bill failed to make it out of committee.[46]

The education program expanded. Short courses began in 1984, which evolved into The Center's famous luncheon lectures. The 1984 fall schedule included "What Should You Be Asking About Your Health?," "Circadian Rhythms, Time Zones and Health," "Smok-

---

42 *Rope*, Dec. 10, 1984.
43 Ibid, January 7, 1985.
44 Ibid, Feb. 4, 1985.
45 Ibid, March 4, 1985.
46 Annual Report 1985, *Rope*.

ing Cessation," "Meeting the Challenge of Change," "Drawing on the Right Side of the Brain," "Communication Through Puppetry," "The Significance of Anaerobic Threshold in Distance Running, Performance and Training," "Using Stress for Your Own Fun and Profit," and "How to Develop a Weight Maintenance Program that Works for You."[47] In 1985, they had such titles as "What Everyone Should Know Before Having Surgery," "Fatigue: The Thief in Our Midst," "How to Be Young at Heart," "Happiness is: Eliminating Unnecessary Depression," and "Do We Really Have to Think About How We Eat and Stuff Like That."[48] The courses used the full range of The Center's staff and consultants.[49] The lectures were just the right thing for the growing self-help movement in the region and throughout the nation.

Then there were tours, something that became a Lewis specialty. There was so much demand for Center tours and there was such an interest among The Center staff in giving a complete and in-depth presentation that it was decided to began charging a modest fee for them. This would eliminate the idle sensation seeker, make it worthwhile to take some time developing a professional tour, and also attract both patients and donors. Lewis was helped by hand-outs and flyers about every element of The Center, linking that piece to the overall mission. The text on the herb garden, for instance, quoted from Henry Beston's *Herbs and the Earth*:

> Peace with the earth is the first peace. Unto so great a mystery, to paraphrase a noble saying, no one path leads, but many paths. What pleasant paths begin in gardens.... The day's high wind is walled off from the herbs, only the taller leaves stirring a little in the fringes of the gusts, the sun mounts from the southeast to the south, the black and yellow bees continue their timeless song. Beautiful and ancient presences of green, dear to us and our human spirit, let us walk awhile beside your leaves."[50]

---

47 Fall courses flyer, 1984, in History Scrapbook #2, CIHF Archives.
48 Activities flyer, n.d. [1985] in ibid.
49 *Rope*, March 4, 1985.
50 Undated flyer [1985], in History Scrapbook #2, CIHF Archives.

While looking at opal, bay laurel, bergamot, cardamom, chamomile, horehound, hyssop, lavender, spiderwort, tansy, tarragon, and yarrow, the visitor absorbed with the fragrance the spirit of the place, and it was that, it was hoped, that would bring the dollars.

A second staff addition in 1985 came in December, when Dr. Jon Sward was hired as Executive Director. Sward had degrees in law (JD) and psychology (PhD), as well as ten years' administrative experience.[51] He was licensed as a minister to boot. At 26 he had become the youngest director of a mental health center in the state of Kansas, and was the first Protestant minister to assist at a Catholic wedding in Kansas in 1967. His interests included guitar, flying, swimming, and writing.[52] He was 41 at the time of his employment at The Center, and Riordan hoped that a long career for Sward would relieve Riordan himself of some of the administrative responsibilities of The Center.[53] Sward came as executive director, but that was not a good fit, so he moved more to patient care in counseling, organized workshops, and after some years opened his own practice.

Research expanded in the new facility. There had long been an ambition for publications, particularly as a way of connecting with the mainstream. Just as The Center was moving into the new facility, the journal *Medical Hypothesis* accepted a research paper from the laboratory entitled "Clinical Correlations Between Serum Glucose Variance and Reported Symptoms in Human Subjects."[54] Late in 1985 research from The Center's lab resulted in a related publication entitled "Differences in Human Serum Copper and Zinc Levels in Healthy and Patient Populations." Three papers were accepted for 1986: "Modulation of Reproduction Output in Drosopilia by Special Properties of Ambient Light" (*Canadian Journal of Zoology*), "Changes in Social Behavior and Brain Catecholamines During the Development of Ascorbate Deficiency in Guinea Pigs" (*Behavioral Process*), and "Behavior and Brain

---

51 *Rope*, Dec. 9, 1985.
52 Staff Profiles, Mabee Library, CIHF.
53 Staff Profiles, Mabee Library, CIHF.
54 *Rope*, Aug. 27, 1984.

Neurotransmitters" (*Behavior and Neural Biology*).

Sometimes Mrs. Garvey was frustrated by the amount of attention paid to research. It was necessary for The Center's tax exempt 501 c (3) status, but it did not bring in income. To the staff, however, it was vital. "These bits of research," the *Rope* reported, "whose titles may sound rather esoteric and removed from the human condition, are in fact providing important knowledge to scientifically support what we know to be true clinically, as we work with patients."[55] All of alternative medicine had been criticized for being "non-scientific" and basing its procedures on anecdotal evidence of cures. Having the science as well as the practice distanced The Center further from those places who had no capacity to explain how and why their patients felt better.[56]

Much of The Center's research, to be sure, was clinical. But some of it was basic bench research. Dr. Phillip Callahan's work, for example, on the biological effects of coherent infrared radiations, had yielded some "startling discoveries."[57] Dr. Callahan in 1985 proposed research that would require about $150,000 in funding for specialized equipment and his residence in Wichita. Callahan's theory was that life processes were controlled by coherent and infrared radiations. "In essence," he said, "life control organic molecules (i.e. sex scents, enzymes, hormones, etc.) emit at room temperature coherent (like radio) infrared emissions that are detected (acted upon) by spines (antenna on insects) and cell structures in all living organisms." Coherent radiation was in phase radiation, not like regular light, which emitted in all directions. The frequencies had to be infrared, since only those short wavelengths would fit the microscopic dimensions of insect and plant spines and human cell walls. Other researchers were beginning to see the potential of this kind of study, but Callahan, having started years ago, was far ahead of them.

Riordan was fascinated by the concept, and The Center very much wanted to support Callahan in what it saw as the kind of potentially

---

55 Ibid, Dec. 2, 1985.
56 Ibid, Sept. 10, 1984.
57 Ibid, Nov. 3, 1986.

Nobel-quality work with which it wished to have an association.[58] Again in 1986, Callahan proposed setting up residence in Wichita and thought that in his first three months working at The Center lab he would create 20 scientific papers.[59] The funding did come from local sources, and Callahan did spend three months in residence at Wichita in the fall of 1986.[60]

There was a fundamental problem, however, with financing the type of research the Garvey Center pursued. Part of it was the feeling among local physicians that The Center was a threat and that its science was flawed. This had led to such rejections of funding requests as that of the Wesley Foundation. But another reason was that much of the research at the Bio-Center lab was not a follow-up on other studies, where considerable momentum and success could be shown in a given direction, nor was it research which could either confirm the effectiveness of or create a profitable product, whether it be a drug, a device, or a procedure. On the contrary, The Center's discoveries often were of the kind that eliminated a profitable drug or treatment in favor of some inexpensive vitamin or nutritional therapy. And it was new. Horace Freeland Judson of Johns Hopkins pointed to that last problem in an article in *Science* in 1986. He wrote: "The grant applications that scientists must submit in order to get their research financed require them to pretend to know what they are going to find out -- Breakthroughs cannot be predicted. What we most want to know about the sciences is thus most securely sealed off from us." The Garvey Center reported that it had felt the "enormous frustration of having grant applications turned down because they dare to truthfully reflect the belief that the discovery of anything non-trivial depends upon unknown contingencies."[61] Ironically for this type of research, there could be no peer review because there were no peers.[62]

---

58 Ibid, July 15, 1985.
59 Ibid, Nov. 3, 1986.
60 Ibid, Dec. 1, 1986.
61 Ibid, Sept. 15, 1986.
62 Ibid, March 23, 1987.

Ironic as it seemed, there was a resistance to effective progress built into the culture. Stanley Davis in his book *Future Perfect* asked why so many things that seemed practical did not happen. His answer was that:

> people have a vested interest in continuing to see time as a restraint, rather than as a resource. By doing so, they have created a role for themselves. People who identify problems generally identify themselves as problem solvers, yet the irony is that they then have a stake in the problem staying identified but unsolved. They adopt the posture that the problem is so large the best they can do is whittle away at it. These people share a common baseline presumption -- the problems are so great that totally eliminating them is an absurd and ridiculous thought!

It was a classic "Catch 22" situation. Those who began to penetrate to the solution were seen as dangerous. "It subverts the context on which the problem solver has built a career, on which the professionals have built their organizations, and on which society has built its institutions."[63]

Generous individual contributions to The Center's research program were a way to get around that insidious inertia. They were the people who "make possible the impossible."[64] Most of the donations to The Center, it reported late in 1986, were in the $25-$50 range. That was a far cry from the $40 million recently left to the Menninger Foundation in Topeka, or the more than $200 million the Wesley Foundation of Wichita had gained from the sale of Wesley Hospital to Hospital Corporation of America in 1985. But, The Center promised to make it go far.[65]

Unlike the large research institutions, the Garvey Center tried to

---

63 Ibid, Feb. 12, 1990.
64 Ibid, Sept. 15, 1986.
65 Ibid, Dec. 8, 1986.

keep in touch with its donors and explain to them the research that it was funding. Those backing Callahan, for instance, received a careful explanation of his research and its significance. "Much of our research is so advanced and on the cutting edge of knowledge that it is difficult to understand." In the case of Callahan, there was a computerized laser device to allow the lab to "see" what was going on in specific infrared frequency ranges. "All life processes at the molecular and cellular level are probably controlled by the emission or absorption of specific infrared frequencies." Most research was done in about one octave of the visible electromagnetic spectrum, but in addition there were eight octaves of microwave emission and 17 of infrared to investigate. "Obviously, the invisible energies in which we are constantly bathed cover enormously wider frequency ranges than do those energies which are visible in the light." The Center was identifying infrared emission and absorption patterns of everything from healthy and sick blood and saliva to nutrients in their raw and processed states. That type of research had never been done before, and the necessary equipment had only recently become available. There was thought of using infrared scanning for the more rapid and complete diagnosis of disease. At the end of this explanation in the *Rope*, there was a response card with a place for the recipient to mark that he did or did not understand the explanation, that he did or did not think this was important research, and that he would or would not like to learn more about research in future communications.[66]

Education was vitally important as the Garvey Center and its peers in alternative medicine continued to come under regular attack. In 1987 there was much media publicity about the use of vitamins, charging that such treatment was experimental and dangerous. The Center responded to its supporters that it was not. "In fact, we simply apply well-known and documented knowledge in the context of understanding that each person is unique biochemically, psychologically and physiologically to help people achieve better health and performance." One of the organizational critics of vitamins was the American Dietetic Association, but

---

66 Ibid, March 23, 1987.

its complaints to the Food and Drug Administration were met by letters from doctors who were "dismayed and angered" that such charges should gain any attention, especially since the ADA was "an organization not known for its scientific acumen and receptivity to new ideas." There was an unfairness about the whole thing, the doctors charged: "The press releases were so deceptive and misleading that it would not be amiss to call them fraudulent." The scientific "experts" included several with "national notoriety for their repeated, shrill and unmeritorious outcries about the supposed harm done by vitamin/mineral consumption." FDA panels should include a range of views. 40% of the US population in 1986 took supplements, yet there had never been a death attributed to them except where doctors had inadvertently overdosed patients with vitamins A and D. And Dr. Donald Davis could find only two documented deaths in the world from vitamin A overdose, one a British PhD chemist who committed suicide by ingesting millions of units. Often mothers called poison control units about a handful of vitamin C tablets a child had taken. But in nearly 25,000 such cases there had never been a death or serious illness. In talking about selenium poisoning the example cited a case where a manufacturer made tablets with 27,000 micrograms instead of the 150 mcg intended. A woman who consumed these mega-tablets had nausea, fatigue and hair loss. It was said she "could have died," but she did not, despite taking a 200 times overdose. The Center in its communications to the FDA asked that agency to ignore the "non-problem" of vitamins and turn its attention to something more serious, like the 130,000 deaths a year in the US from the use of prescription drugs.[67]

The Center did have one threatened lawsuit in 1986 about vitamin A. A woman, after being treated there and marrying an attorney, sent a letter threatening to sue for $50,000 and The Center's malpractice insurance carrier, much to Dr. Riordan's chagrin, settled for $3,000. Riordan wrote the insurance company: "In my opinion, it is because of such short-term benefit approaches (let us get rid of the threat of a lawsuit as cheaply as possible) that we are in the malpractice quagmire

---

67 Ibid, Feb. 9, 1987.

that exists today. When a potential suit is without merit, as this one is, I believe that we need to bow our necks and say no. The only compensation I would offer would be based on our Center's policy which has always been to refund payment to a person who was dissatisfied with our services."[68]

The ongoing insurance controversy was another burden to bear. That had been dormant for a time as The Center concentrated on its move, but in 1987 a father threatened to sue the insurance company after his health insurance company refused payment for treatment by the Garvey Center. The company had paid more than $20,000 for two years of outpatient and hospital care for the man's daughter elsewhere without result, and then refused The Center's modest fee when it had effected dramatic improvement.

The father's threats generated inquiries from the insurance company, to which Riordan responded. He sent an entire box of articles dealing with the biochemistry of depression as it related to people like this patient. As a check The Center inserted little threads to determine whether the material was ever opened. A letter from the insurance people said they had read the material thoroughly and rejected the claim, but on the return of the box the threads were intact. [69]

Riordan explained that because of the patient's low level of the essential, sulfur-containing amino acid Methionine during her initial exam, the relation between amino acid metabolism and depression were the focus of the care. The relation between hypoascorbemia and depression had been noted in every standard medical textbook for 30 years, and Riordan did not see why The Center's approach to the case should be controversial.

> From my perspective as a clinician who sees only people who have been treated medically elsewhere without success, I find your request for information supporting what we do to be most frustrating, albeit standard. What

---

68 Ibid, April, 9, May 12, 1986.
69 Interview, Dr. Hugh Riordan with Craig Miner, October 22, 1998.

you should be interested in when deciding whether to pay a bill for one of your insured is how they do— what kind of result they are having. Instead you pay for process however dismal the outcome may be. As the result, you pay enormous amounts for established but ineffective processes because they are the accepted thing to do instead of paying for what works in this case. As a consequence, countless people suffer because physicians, in part coerced by reimbursable insurance payments, find it easier to 'do things right' than doing the right thing.

Someday, Riordan thought, there would be a class action suit for fraud against insurance companies that did not provide insurance.[70]

The issue came up again in 1989 when a new physician at The Center, Dr. Ronald Hunninghake, took over the mantle from others to add new energy to the battle. Hunninghake had served an internship at Wesley in 1978 and at that time ran across a notice on a bulletin board for one of The Center's international conferences. He attended, saw the model of the Master Facility there, and, like so many others, thought to himself "that will never happen." After beginning practice in Salina, he went to a Holistic Medicine Association meeting in Wisconsin and met Riordan again there. He developed a wellness program in his family practice office in Salina and found patients responded well to it, physically and emotionally. But he was frustrated by the time crunch. Not only did he personally have little time for his young family, being on call all hours of the day and night, but little time for his patients.

Philosophically, the practice did not seem quite to fit. Hunninghake was certified as a transcendental meditation instructor. He had been a vegetarian and was a serious runner, having competed in two marathons. He believed strongly in what one author called "Positive Addictions," yet was experiencing stress right along with the high income from standard medical practice. Moving was a risk, telling his partners was difficult, but Hunninghake did it, and became "Dr. Ron" of The Center.

---

70 *Rope*, April 8, 20, 1987.

The transition, even then, was slow, and Hunninghake commuted the 90 miles from Salina for the first year and a half he worked in Wichita. He found it, however, deeply satisfying, and noticed that there never was a day any more when he dreaded coming to work. He no longer saw himself as a "rescuer," but as a helper, and it made a large difference. "You have to live it, do it, and experience it," he said.[71] Certainly his presence at last relieved Riordan of some of the responsibility of day to day patient care and put The Center on a broader footing.[72]

The synergism between Hunninghake and Riordan was excellent. Riordan was the diagnostician and both he and Hunninghake were detectives in the quest to discover underlying reasons for the patient/co-learner's illnesses. Riordan continued to see all patients first, but then many of their remaining contacts were with Hunninghake. Hunninghake was energetic, kind, spiritual, an excellent speaker, and a great enthusiast for The Center. He had a great sense of humor and was quickly perceived to live the life that he recommended to others. So focused was he that once his wife came home from a trip, having asked Dr. Ron to stay home and watch the kids, to find him with his laptop on a card table in the middle of the yard working on a speech with not a child to be seen. Staff noted that "everyone feels comfortable with him." He seemed genuinely interested in everyone, which was exactly a fit with the philosophy of The Center.[73] In the year 2000 Hunninghake's title was Medical Director of the Olive Garvey Center for Healing Arts.

Hunninghake emphasized in a 1989 letter to the members of the Pathology Liaison Committee of Blue Cross and Blue Shield of Kansas that he was a graduate of the University of Kansas Medical School and was certified by the American Board of Family Practice. He addressed the concerns the insurance industry seemed to have about The Center and The Center's responses. First, what was the appropriate relationship between an insurance company and a medical care facility "which

---

71 Interview, Dr. Ron Hunninghake with Craig Miner, November 18, 1998.
72 Interview, Dr. Hugh Riordan with Craig Miner, October 22, 1998.
73 Interview, Laura Benson and Marilyn Landreth with Craig Miner, Aug. 19, 1999.

is staffed by licensed and certified medical doctors, where the focus of services offered to patients has a unique character?" It seemed obvious there should be some appropriate relationship. Second, did it not benefit insurance subscribers with "complicated multifactorial illnesses" who had not responded to standard diagnosis and treatment to find satisfaction and help elsewhere? Third, given current public interest in nutrition with strong demand that it be applied to the medical setting, did not an alliance between insurance companies and The Center make sense? Fourth, modern medical care was an "acute reactive paradigm" with best success in care of infectious disease and trauma. But the majority of illnesses were chronic. As the population aged, there would be more of them, and the care, without early intervention, would be "end-stage, palliative, and very, very expensive." Was that a good outcome? Fifth, the Garvey Center was uniquely situated to take care of such people. "The focus of treatment is not on one specific diagnosis, one disease, or even one lab abnormality. Rather, the biochemical basis of multiple interacting metabolic imbalances that underlie the various symptom and disease processes are uncovered with a thorough laboratory analysis." Was that not a rational approach? Sixth, results were satisfactory to patient and doctor, and there were no problems at The Center with iatrogenic (physician-induced) disease. The Center was starting a six year study to determine if patients who had gone through its approach became low cost utilizers of standard medical care. It was thought they did. Seventh, it seemed there was a "defined subset of patients" just suited to The Center, and they should be there. "The vicious and expensive downward spiral of chronic illness is broken with a comprehensive, highly personal approach where the biochemical foundations of the patient's disabilities are identified and rationally treated in the context of proper lifestyle and optimal health." Hunninghake hoped his seven points would serve as the basis for a "new dialogue" with the insurance companies. "These are difficult times in the field of medical care. I would hope that a spirit of innovation would not be dashed on the rocks of short-sighted crisis management."[74]

---

74 Letter, Ron Hunninghake to Blue Cross, Nov. 10, 1989, in History Scrapbook #3, CIHF Archives.

There seemed again to be some movement. Riordan said to the state insurance commissioner at Topeka that "if we are to reduce the enormous, burgeoning cost of sickness care, we must have the insurance industry pay for what works."[75] And in January 1989 Riordan appeared before insurance commissioner Fletcher Bell and his staff. Riordan told them he wanted a meeting with representatives of the carriers to try to reach a position of "common sense." He thought a "reasonable goal" was that whenever insured people stipulated that their condition had been improved and that they were satisfied with their care, and so long as that care generated fees that were less than those that were paid by insurance carriers to those people for less effective procedures, their claims should be ordered paid by the Kansas Insurance Commissioner. Bell listened politely, but said he did not know that he had the power to do that.[76]

The next month there was a meeting of the senior counsel and staff of some insurance companies. They explained their reasons for not paying for good results. Dr. Jon Sward suggested that the discussion would get further if the group discussed mutual interests rather than defending positions already adopted. Did all not wish to reduce the cost of medical care and did not all wish that patients got well? One Blue Cross representative did state that "alternative approaches to sickness should be reviewed because throughout the history of medicine, it has been those doing nonstandard things that have prompted the profession to advance."[77] However, the meetings brought no breakthroughs. Frustration resumed in Wichita, and the mail was not heavy with insurance checks for the Garvey Center.

Such controversies emphasized the need for education and for a public presence. In the summer of 1986 The Center held an "I Like Wichita" contest. Kansans and Wichitans had an inferiority complex, it was widely believed, yet there was no good reason for it. "Because our Center has already had the pleasure of serving people from all 50 states

---

75 *Rope*, Oct. 24, 1988.
76 Ibid, Jan. 9, 1989.
77 Ibid, Feb. 6, 1989.

and 12 foreign countries," CIHF publicity noted, "we know how most visitors who come here feel about Wichita. They like it. At the same time, we know that there is an almost institutionalized negativity or at least a downplay of what is good about our city when Wichitans talks with our counterparts in other areas of the country. For economic development to flourish, the ratio of positive self-image to negative self-image must increase to a more realistic level." Consequently The Center offered a grand prize of $1,000 and four runner-up prizes of $250 for essays on why people liked Wichita. The prizes were doubled if the entrants had taken a tour of The Center and had their entry blanks stamped.[78] Entry forms were distributed through Dillon's food stores, and the essays were judged that fall by a local panel.[79]

The contest received much favorable publicity locally, though *Eagle* columnist Bob Goetz wondered why the sponsoring institution had one of the "longest and most unfathomable names of any business ever hatched.... Whatever happened to simple names like Olive's, huh?"[80]

The contest pleased the staff because it fitted The Center's philosophy. Riordan responded to a negative article about Wichita in the newspaper by noting that "the writer provides the usual litany in which we're supposed to whip ourselves because we are not Kansas City, Chicago, Dallas, or Denver. Neither are we London, Tokyo or Vienna. We are Wichita." As citizens, it seems, we had the same problems as people had with their health. They were trying to fit into some standard model instead of appreciating local uniqueness. "As any sculptor knows," Riordan commented, "a work of art does not come about by cursing the block of wood or lump of clay because they are not things of beauty. The work of art comes about because the sculptor perceives the beauty within the block of wood or lump of clay and gradually chips away or forms and shapes it until that vision of a thing of beauty becomes a reality."[81]

---

78 Ibid, July 14, 1986. *Wichita Eagle Beacon*, Sept. 10, 1986, History Scrapbook #2, CIHF Archives.
79 *Rope*, Oct. 13, 1986.
80 *Wichita Eagle Beacon*, Sept. 10, 1986, History Scrapbook #2, CIHF Archives.
81 Letter, Hugh Riordan to Editor, in *Wichita Eagle Beacon*, Sept. 6, 1986, ibid.

Riordan spoke in June 1987 to the Entrepreneurship Camp at Wichita State University about his methods. "We are practicing medicine today," he told the group, "as it will be practiced in the year 2000 by the majority of physicians." Because The Center was on the leading edge, it was the equivalent of an entrepreneurial enterprise in business. But it was hardly any longer, by any measure, total quackery. The American Cancer Society and the National Cancer Institute had by 1987 recognized the link between diet and cancer, and the American Heart Association had long recognized the link between diet and cardiovascular disease. The Arthritis Foundation still insisted, however that what people ate had no bearing on how well their joints functioned, and a diabetes organization recently provided candy for people to take when contributing their change to the fight against the disease. The public was wiser than some of the professionals, and Riordan's recommendations were MYBA (Move your Body Around), EWF (Eat Wholesome Food), and TST (Think Stimulating Thoughts).[82]

The Center's Bio-Communications Press was another educational outreach. It published its first book in 1987 — Roger Williams' *The Wonderful World Within You*. In 1988 came Emanuel Cheraskin's *The Vitamin C Controversy: Questions and Answers*, Carl Pfeiffer's *The Schizophrenias: Ours To Conquer*, and volume one of *Medical Mavericks* by Dr. Hugh Riordan. In 1989 the press published Cheraskin's *Health and Happiness*, along with *Hypnosis, Acupuncture & Pain*, by Dr. Maurice Tinterow, *Medical Mavericks*, vol. 2 by Riordan and two editions of *From the Heart*, a cookbook by Nanda Langston, Beverly Kindel, and Regina Miller.

Barbara Nichols in May 1986 answered an ad in the newspaper that said "We're looking for someone who loves to type," with a return address with no company name or phone number. The job was Publishing Coordinator for The Center's Bio-Communications Press, and Barbara became an expert not only in word processing, but in the then-new field of desktop publishing using The Center's Apple MacIntosh computers. The books were advertised in a remarkable new Center

---

82 *Rope*, June 8, 1987.

publication edited by Richard Lewis and called *Health Hunters*.[83] Olive Garvey, who so seldom mixed in the everyday decision-making, suggested that name.[84]

Health Hunters originated in 1986 as the name of a membership program with The Center for the public and for employees of corporations.[85] This service was advertised on television.[86]

The first issue of the *Health Hunters* newsletter, produced by The Center's desk top computer publishing operation, appeared in April 1987. Richard Lewis wrote most of the text, with Arline Magnusson contributing the "Superb Herb" section and Marilyn Landreth describing the books and tapes that The Center had for sale.[87] Among those sale items in the first issue were *The Relaxed Body Book*, a cassette called *The Sky of Mind*, and a guide to *Bio-Nutrionics: Lower Your Cholesterol in 30 Days*. There were quotations from Leonardo da Vinci and Epictetus, and considerable statistics on health.[88] Other issues that first year hawked Manheim Steamroller tapes, Zamfir meditations and, Holly Atkinson's book *Women and Fatigue* and offered to send a kit to introduce people to Dr. Burkitt's "floaters" club. But the key element of the newsletter was the ever more sophisticated feature called "Just for the Health of It" and the pieces reprinted from the press all over the world.

"No one can expect to live long if he disregards the nature of his environment," said the lead article for the July/August 1987 issue, "--if he remains naked and unsheltered when a blizzard blows, if he travels unprotected under the desert sun, if he stands his ground when a hurricane approaches. Persons who disregard the quality of their food environment are behaving in the same foolhardy way." All human beings, all earthly organisms share an underlying biochemical unity. Therefore all lives are interwoven and "nature is on our side. This is not

---

83 Ibid, June 29, 1987. "My Thoughts about The Center," by Barbara Nichols (c. 1998), Office Files, CIHF Archives.
84 Interview, Dr. Hugh Riordan to Craig Miner, October 22, 1998.
85 *Rope*, April 14, June 9, 1986.
86 Ibid, June 30, 1986.
87 Ibid, Feb. 25, 1988.
88 *Health Hunter*, vol. 1, no. 1 (April, 1987), CIHF Archives.

a world in which good internal environments are unattainable.... Our fundamental task is to understand nature and learn to live with it and be a part of it." [89]

That level of insight was typical, and with it went hard-hitting factual information. Other members of the staff and consultants began contributing to communicate their sometimes esoteric fields of expertise to a lay audience and to suggest practical ways in which that audience could use that knowledge to improve their health and their lives.[90] Marv Dirks wrote in February 1988. "Adapting to the tough times in life is something we all have to do," he wrote. "The more strength and energy we have to deal with life, the more satisfying we find it." Norepinephrine and serotonin levels could be changed by diet for good or ill and moods would follow apace. Coffee and cigarettes damaged here as well as in so many other ways. The same issue contained "cold facts about cold cuts." Bologna could have 90 calories per oz. with 84% of them coming from fat, and throwing in 300 mgs. of sodium. Cuts claiming to be 95% fat free had that figure calculated by weight not calories. 35% of the calories could still be fat.[91] The April 1988 issue contained practical advice on getting cholesterol under 200 without drugs, introducing most Wichita readers for the first time to Essential Fatty Acids (EFAs) and their use.[92] That fall, readers learned the difference between Aging and Getting Old. Getting Old was inevitable, but "effective adaptation minimizes the destructive, entropic changes of aging and promotes the full development and growth of the individual." It was necessary that aging readers be "responsible health hunters rather than helpless illness victims" and design their environments according to their needs.[93] There was also an article that fall on Chinese medicine by Dr. Tinterow and one by Dr. Callahan on what we can learn from the "insignificant insect." The "Superb Herb" docu-

---

89 Ibid, vol. 1, no. 4 (July/Aug., 1987).
90 Ibid, vol. 1, no. 6 (Oct., 1987).
91 Ibid, vol. 2, no. 2 (Feb., 1988).
92 Ibid, vol. 2, no. 4 (April, 1988).
93 Ibid, vol. 2, no. 8 (Sept. 1988).

mented what was meant by someone's "feeling his oats." Before the general oat bran craze, The Center noted that oats were easily digested, had been used as a nerve tonic, anti-spasmodic and anti-depressant, could prevent wrinkles, were excellent for bowel regulation, while their soluble fiber helped control blood sugar, even in diabetics, and lowered total cholesterol. Why not try oatmeal for breakfast?[94]

Health Hunters was filled with the kind of innovative statements that were The Center's specialty, but they were never without documentation, nor without a suggestion about how bad situations could be changed. In 1989, it was pointed out that the angry and cynical were five times more likely to die before age 50 than others, and that fast-talking type-A attorneys were at special risk. "Trusting hearts last longer because they are protected from the ravages of the sympathetic nervous system."[95] Wisdom was communicated from Plato, Hippocrates, Socrates, and the Spanish Jewish philosopher Moses Maimonides. And there was advice on the best choices if one had to dine on fast foods.[96] It was a significant addition to The Center's educational program and remained a prominent feature of its outreach. *Health Hunter* members got discounts on purchases at The Center and they got a very interesting and well-designed publication every month.

The international conferences continued. The 9th one, held in September 1985, was catered by the in-house kitchen staff and videotaped with The Center's own equipment.[97] Conference 10 in September 1987 included Dr. Bjorksten on "Longevity, Past-Present-Future;" Dr. Donald Davis speaking on "Differential Nutrition -- a New Orientation From Which to Approach the Problems of Human Nutrition;" Paul Lee, PhD on "The Biological Basis of the History of Consciousness;" and Dr. Spears on "Energy Cycles in the Body."[98] Over 300 people attended that year.[99] The 11th conference included Dr. Joseph Beas-

---

94 Ibid, vol. 2, no. 9 (Oct., 1988), vol. 2, no. 10 (Nov., 1988).
95 Ibid, vol. 3, no. 2 (Feb., 1989).
96 Ibid, vol. 3, no. 9 (Oct., 1989).
97 *Rope*, September 16, 1985.
98 Program in History Scrapbook #3, CIHF Archives.
99 *Rope*, Feb. 25, 1988.

ley's "Wrong Diagnosis, Wrong Treatment" on alcoholism; Dr. Walter Blumer on "Cancer Prevention by Chelation Therapy;" Dae Chang, PhD on "Dietary Determinism" in criminals; Dr. Hunninghake on "The New Medicine: Medical Care in the 21st Century;" and Vernon Woolf, PhD on "Viewing the Mind as a Holodigm."[100] Attendance at that conference was limited to 120 by the facilities used, but was evaluated by Riordan as "the best we have ever held." The electronic recording was flawless and the "Taste of Health" catering staff got a standing ovation. The Center had in place an ambitious and well-integrated program to spread the word. Riordan wrote Olive Garvey that "I trust you realize the enormity of the positive impact The Center is having on the lives of many, many people — and will have in the future through our research, services to patients, and educational efforts. I believe we are on the verge of becoming internationally recognized for our excellence in all three areas."[101]

There remained a financial challenge as Mrs. Garvey cut back her support. The Center kept approaching foundations, but largely without success, mainly because the research was so innovative. One example was a request for funding from the Markey Charitable Trust in 1986 for infrared research. The proposal, which Riordan thought was one of the best he had ever written, was first reviewed by a surgeon at Stanford. His rejection message was "that infrared had nothing to do with anything." Of course, he had no awareness that people existed in one octave of visible light and 17 octaves of infrared.[102] But there were increasing donations from individuals who had been patients, and there was the prospect of the fee and sales income sustaining the operation. In the spring of 1986 came an interesting possibility from a group of people in Oregon who had a remarkable stock of over 3,500 varieties of herb seeds, were interested in The Center's lab facilities, and were "willing basically to work at the poverty level and share in the proceeds of gardening and seed sales."

---

100 Ibid, Sept., 1989.
101 Letter, Riordan to Olive Garvey, Sept. 25, 1989, Office Files, CIHF Archives.
102 Ibid, Jan. 3, 1986. Interview, Dr. Hugh Riordan with Craig Miner, Feb. 1, 2000.

The problem for Riordan was that, although they were brilliant (the staff included the youngest person ever to get a PhD from Yale) they looked and dressed like hippies.[103] Already Riordan had developed a "maverick index" to determine "if research people wanting to work here have the intestinal fortitude to stand the criticism that comes our way."[104] Riordan was hopeful. "I can't even imagine what my life would have been like," he wrote at the 11th anniversary of The Center in the fall of 1986, "had we not had that fateful meeting in your office with Cliff Allison, Carl Pfieffer and Bill Schul in the spring of 1975. The miracle that that meeting generated has already touched the lives of over ten thousand patients and participants in our health-related programs." By the year 2000, Riordan hoped "to be able to list many, many scientific accomplishments and to say that I have devoted more than a third of my life to help make The Center the reality it is. But, we have to get there from here."[105]

The thinking was intense, with many brain-storming sessions among the staff. "As you and I both know," Riordan wrote to Garvey early in 1987, "although we have 40 plus staff members, The Center's basic energy is generated by Hugh Riordan. This is primarily because I am the only one who has had the clear long-term commitment to making The Center a reality and a force in the medical-health field." He was also the only one willing "to risk my professional status on the rise and fall of The Center without any guarantees financial or otherwise." But he would like others in that boat with him to create more "balance and future continuity." To do that he wanted more than year-to-year funding from Garvey in order to attract more cautious physicians. "I suspect that you are tired of hearing of our needs as I see them. In the current scheme of things in which we as yet have been unable to secure large-scale funding from typical non-visionary foundations, I find it necessary to communicate with the one person who has the greatest vision of all."[106] He visited Garvey in Scottsdale and attended to her

---

103 Letter, Riordan to Olive Garvey, April 16, 1986, CIHF Office Files.
104 Ibid, Aug. 12, 1986.
105 Ibid, Oct. 24, 1986.
106 Ibid, March 31, 1987.

health needs. "I do not *want* to live *forever*," she told him, "but I like to be comfortable and as active as possible as long as I can."[107]

There was a substantial exchange of long letters between Garvey and Riordan in August 1987 about finances and about operations — a struggle at a crossroads in many ways. Riordan started the exchange with an 11-page missive on August 9 that responded to Bob Page's suggestions about a need for restructuring at The Center. Since Page was the Garvey family's most trusted advisor and a substantial supporter of The Center financially in his own right, such a "suggestion" was not to be ignored.

One idea coming from the Garvey building was that by adding more doctors, The Center could realize more income from direct services similar to those it now performed. Profits from there could support other areas that would never be self-sufficient. "There is no question," Riordan responded, "that we need more doctors, that we want more of them and that we shall have more doctors." However, a review of the situation revealed some complicating factors. First, it was a new day and age, and the medical profession, with the exception of surgery, was not so highly cost effective as formerly. Second, The Center's fees were too low to make the clinical division produce great income. Third, there was "a limited population base" who believed in The Center's approach. "The lengthy process needed by people to gain information, change their medical belief system and then change their medically related behavior precludes a great stampede to our door." Fourth, there was the insurance company refusal to reimburse.

Some things could be changed that might help. The basic fee could be raised from $75 to $100 an hour. That would make adding physicians profitable, provided that they could be kept busy seeing patients most of the time. But as fees rose some patients were priced out. Even with extensive publicity, Riordan could not see adding more than one physician a year over the next three years. Another option on fees would be to "massively increase" them to the level of some practitioners in the country who were charging "from $1,000 to say hello to $15,000 for a

---

107 Letter, Olive Garvey to Riordan, April 10, 1987, Office Files, CIHF Archives.

one week evaluation." But, he concluded "such an approach would be philosophically incongruent with our mission to help as many people as possible."

The lab was not doing as well financially as in the early years, partly because of the change in insurance practice. That had led the lab's previously strong referral business from physicians around the country to decline. "They simply don't order tests insurance doesn't pay for because they don't want irate patients on their hands." It appeared that the lab would have to get half its funding from research endowments.

The educational outreach was working well. Fees for it could be increased, and more books could be published. But that was not likely to be a major source of income so much as a source of good public relations.

Other possibilities were problematic, too. Riordan did not feel comfortable allowing large donors to name board members. It would interfere with the independence that was such a feature of The Center. However, The Center had reached a $2,000,000 endowment level, and that would take some of the pressure off Garvey for yearly support of research.

There was the suggestion that the name of The Center be changed. Riordan wrote that he was aware of the merits of that but "I would find it difficult to continue to be personally involved if that was done. After all, this Center exists only because of you. I would rather go down in flames treasuring your vision, your support and your name than succumb to what we fight daily in the medical world — namely doing things right rather than doing the right thing." But, there was the possibility of pleasing everyone. Perhaps the Olive Garvey name could be retained for that part of The Center that directly dealt with people and the research arm could be called something else.

The long letter closed with another suggestion, which Riordan said was "both very selfish on my part and possibly the best way to perpetuate what The Center stands for as we approach the year 2000." That was to create a Hugh Riordan lifetime endowment of one million dollars to enable him to pursue research interests to enhance human functioning. The principal would never be touched and would revert to Garvey interests upon Riordan's death. It would allow him, after the physicians were trained, "to be a much more potent spokesman for

The Center approach. And I would have the security that my livelihood could not be destroyed by the state board revoking my license to practice medicine." Such an endowment would reduce The Center's operational expense by the amount of Riordan's salary, and "short of death, it would represent the greatest change that could occur in my professional life."[108]

Olive responded at length. Maybe she had been wrong wanting to keep lab prices so low anyone could afford them. "Direct services of value should generate commensurate income. They are worth their keep. People generally appreciate things which cost them …. Business is business and charity is charity and never the twain will mix." The TV production had been the first departure from the straight and narrow. That was "ingenious and very valuable," but not profitable. The Master Facility was perhaps too big for current needs and too innovative ever to sell easily. "Next you went into the restaurant business, this too, partly educational of nutrition, partly publicity." But it was a money loser. Now The Center was into printing, with financial results unknown. And Riordan was trying to do it all:

> As everyone acknowledges, you and you alone, are the adhesive which holds all of this together. As everyone knows, you, like all of us, are mortal. The reason some of the above enterprises have not succeeded as you wished is because you have tried to economize on capability of employees, and you, yourself, are spread too thin. You *cannot* do it *alone*. Besides you could 'be hit by a truck' today. No institution should depend for its stability on one man.

The Garvey Foundation had contributed to The Center millions of dollars, and it was time to protect its investment. Olive had several requests. She supposed The Center had a constitution. She thought the board should be increased to seven or nine and that Olive should approve

---

108 Letter, Riordan to Olive Garvey, August 9, 1987, ibid.

one more than half of them. The Center should have a manager, a professional public relations department or a contract with a firm, rather than using "less capable amateurs." There should be a woman's auxiliary. The Center should hire two new doctors before January 1, 1988, and three before January 1, 1989. It should hire a professional fund-raiser before January 1, 1989. And it should change its name. The name was too long, Olive said, and the organization would have better luck raising funds without her name on it. "My own reaction to Frank Carney and Charles Koch when they ask for funds for something is, 'let them do it.' I think that reaction exists about The Center." The name, she thought, should emphasize research: "That will give it stature and create more sympathy."

Again, too, she re-emphasized her limits. "You have an exaggerated idea about all of those millions you are suggesting I extend. They are distinctly limited and some are committed elsewhere. If I dip into capital it is 'killing the goose which lays the golden eggs,' and that I am *not* willing to do." The dreams would have to fit the funding. "In the long run I have been very proud and pleased with what you have accomplished. Probably the dissenters would not tell *me*, but people have ventured many, many positive reports. I believe wholeheatedly in what you are doing and want to help to the extent of my ability."[109]

Out of this strain, even almost agony, of thinking, came, instead of stagnation or dispirit, remarkable and original initiatives. Late in the 1980s emerged two great Center initiatives identified by what became familiar acronyms to Center staff and supporters: ABNA and RECNAC. Both projects had startling premises. The first was that The Center would treat patients unable to find help elsewhere for no charge at the time of service. They would be asked to contribute for 6 years, according to how well they did and their means. The second was that it would discover the causes of cancer within ten years.

ABNA stood for "Achievable Benefits Not Achieved," a term coined by Dr. Williamson when he was at Johns Hopkins. The premise was radical. Why not make The Center an entirely research institution, working with a limited number of persons as patients who could be

---

109 Letter, Olive Garvey to Riordan, Aug. 14, 1987, ibid.

helped, but had not been helped? Mrs. Garvey could provide funding for their care as part of a contribution to the research operation, and then the patients themselves would contribute to The Center whatever amount they wished based on the benefit to them. This system would eliminate considerable billing and time keeping, and it might be the case that gratitude would result in more money than a fee schedule.

Riordan, writing about this idea to Page in December 1987, called it "my best Sunday evening shot at presenting either the craziest con-job or the greatest stroke of genius of my medical career. Only time will tell which." There would be a one-time fee of $100 to apply for the program. If 10,000 people applied, that by itself would bring in $1 million. Those not accepted would get a nutritional profile worth $100 retail and a packet of other materials. "In my opinion the potential is absolutely astounding. The question is will potential be translated into bottom line success?"[110]

The possibilities would, he thought, be similar to venture capital operations in which 1/3 were expected to lose money, 1/3 be neutral, and 1/3 bring in big money. Riordan had experimented a few years earlier with giving free care to three patients, and that was the pattern there: one gave nothing, one about the cost of the care, and the third a substantial amount. By providing free research-based care The Center also would "insure IRS friendliness in the future, protecting all giving to date; would greatly enhance the likelihood of receiving real and personal property tax exemptions and would enormously increase our gut level appeal to attract contributors." Olive could give $1 million for matching to start this.[111] Certainly ABNA would take all restraints off the kind of care The Center wished to give. It would allow the doctors to focus on just one goal: helping the person achieve maximum benefits. "They no longer need be concerned that they cannot get a complete testing profile because the patient cannot afford it or the insurance company will not pay for it."[112]

---

110 Letter, Riordan to Robert Page, Dec. 6, 1987, ibid.
111 Letter from Riordan, n.d., ibid.
112 *Rope*, Feb. 25, 1988.

ABNA opened in April 1988 and operated for one year. It got considerable publicity, including praise from a local doctor who said of Riordan: "He needs to do this. If he can get a thousand people and monitor them over a significant period of time, he will establish credulity."[113] There was a large public relations program for it, but The Center received only hundreds of applications, not the 10,000 it had planned. Contributions from the patients provided over $60,000 to the research funding the first year, but it was not sufficient to make The Center self-sustaining.[114]

It did much, however, to help The Center's reputation. George Neavoll of the *Wichita Eagle* visited right at the end of the ABNA experiment as a guest of Dr. Maurice Tinterow, who was starting a third career just then as a Center physician. They dined on buffalo at the Taste of Health restaurant, and Neavoll commented that The Center was a unique facility. "While Wichitans slept, it took form and shape, and now is on the edge of breakthroughs in clinical research and holistic health so significant they could alter the course of human history." Tinterow, a man with both an MD and PhD who had spent 40 years as an anesthesiologist and six years as a professor at WSU, was typical of the people one found at the domes along Chisholm Creek. So was Riordan. "Defying all the 'rules' of the profession," Neavoll wrote of The Center's founder, "he follows whatever he thinks the truth might be, regardless of where that may be. He delights in deflating the egos of the pompous, and considers his patients his equals."[115] Another reporter, visiting from Houston, evaluated Riordan in a similar way: "He doesn't look or sound like a kook. Riordan stands about 6-foot-3 inches and is built like a plow horse. He looks like a farmer. Or a former pro football linebacker. He speaks simply and sensibly." And, he was experimenting with giving free health care. It got peoples' attention.[116]

Still, it was not the be all and end all. There was no financial magic.

---

113 Unidentified clipping in History Scapbook #3, CIHF Archives.
114 Annual Report 1988 in *Rope*.
115 *Wichita Eagle Beacon*, Aug. 20, 1989, History Scrapbook #2, CIHF Archives.
116 Kathleen Myler in *Houston Chronicle*, n.d. [1989], ibid.

"I sympathize with your enthusiasm," Olive wrote in the fall of 1988, "but your timetable may be overly ambitious." She estimated she had contributed substantially greater millions of dollars to what began as a lab project at a budget of about $100,000. "I know research must be subsidized and I have done most of that. You are going to *have to find* support from a *wider range* than Garvey and Page. Every well runs dry." Doing that, she understood, would be "the greatest challenge of your career.... But I cannot carry it alone and I think it may require more time than you wish."[117]

RECNAC was "Cancer" spelled backward. Officially it stood for "Research Encompassing Comprehensive Novel Approaches to Cancer."[118] The name was suggested by one of The Center's long-term cancer survivors, Zelma Barrackman, a public health nurse, because she said that our goal was to reverse the incidence and death rate from cancer.[119] The initial funding came from Bob Page. The press release announcing it came on February 9, 1989. The Center's research division, it said, would undertake a "time limited, highly goal-oriented research thrust" backed by a vision that "goes a tad beyond what is usual, ordinary, or standard." It would try to raise $20 million for discovering the cause of cancer, a drop-in-the-bucket compared to the funds already devoted to such research, but unprecedented for the Wichita organization.

Cancer had been studied intensively in the US for forty years without any real breakthrough. The number of deaths from all cancers had, in fact, grown since 1970. It was the "plague of the 20th century," affecting one in four Americans. It might seem ridiculous that such a small place as the OWGCIHF ("our small, ragtag research group" Riordan called it) should undertake to study such a large problem, since "it is apparently so complicated and because so many great minds have tried to find the answers without success." Yet some chance observations in the lab, and some success with cancer patients had stimulated the Wichita researchers to think real progress was possible in their shop. Therefore

---

117 Letter, Olive Garvey to Riordan, Oct. 25, 1988, ibid.
118 *Wichita Eagle*, July 15, 1992, History Scrapbook #4, CIHF Archives.
119 Interview, Dr. Hugh Riordan with Craig Miner, October 22, 1998.

The Center announced that on February 9, 1999 (later extended to December 31, 1999), it would report on how and why cancer occurs in living organisms, and would thus in a magnificent way kick off its 25th anniversary celebration. Or else, it would admit defeat and move out of the way for others. There was a chance. Roger Bacon had said once that "more secrets of knowledge have been discovered by plain and neglected men than by men of popular fame. And this is so with reason. For the men of popular fame are busy on popular matters."[120]

Reaction was mixed, probably a bit on the contemptuous side nationally. The media contacted the National Cancer Institute, which opined that the project was foolishness because no one was going to find the answer to cancer; it was too complex. Riordan said later that he wondered why then the nation was spending 1.5 billion tax dollars a year on cancer research. Would the space program have been funded if the notion had been that it was nice to get into space, but obviously we could not do it?[121] John Lough of the American Institute for Cancer research said: "My initial reaction, obviously is one of some confusion. It's not the sort of disease that lends itself out to timetables and budget constraints.... It does not sound realistic at all." Riordan replied: "I don't think what we do is wacky. We use good, sound techniques to achieve good results. I'm sure many people think it's a grandiose notion and impossible to accomplish, but time will tell.... I would think 99% of the people would think it's out of this world." The Center at the time of the announcement had a $500,000 grant from Bob Page for the project, and a projected total operating budget of $2 million a year. The American Cancer Society's annual budget was $300 million. The National Cancer Institute, the nation's government-funded clearing-house for cancer research, had an annual budget to $1.6 billion.[122]

Riordan had been looking through his microscope and thinking

---

120 Media News Release from Bio-Communications Research Institute, Feb. 9, 1989, History Scrapbook #3, CIHF Archives.
121 Interview, Dr. Hugh Riordan with Craig Miner, October 22, 1998.
122 "Olive Garvey Center Shugs off Skeptics, Begins Cancer Research," *Wichita Eagle Beacon*, Feb. 9, 1989, ibid.

about the differences in the behavior of cells in the darkness of the body and away from electromagnetic interference compared with the way they behaved in ordinary labs.[123] He had treated several cancer patients, beginning with a dentist who was suffering from cancer of the pancreas and had become interested in The Center's work through attending one of its international conferences. The dentist called in October, said that he was supposed to be dead by Thanksgiving, and made the simple request to Riordan to try to keep him alive long enough to go on his annual ski trip over Christmas. The Center put him on what it would later consider relatively small doses of intravenous vitamin C, under 15 grams a week. He skied that winter and the next. The second February, he asked to be taken off the vitamin therapy, was, and died in July. There were even some cases where a cancer with extensive metastasis went away entirely. That could have been a coincidence, but Riordan could hardly ignore the promise.

The C therapy, a kind of "natural chemotherapy," suited him far better than the drastic measures being taken in standard medicine using toxic chemicals against the disease. He had watched his consultant Dr. Spears suffer from uterine cancer, and even more, it seemed, from the treatment of it, and thought there must be a better way. "I seriously doubt," he said, "that chemotherapy will be around long. It will be viewed like bloodletting in fifty years. If the part offends you, get rid of it one way or the other. I think it is time now to move on to the New Testament. It is a very punishing experience. That would be alright if you just want to get punished, but it is pretty devastating." And he was willing to act on his intuition.[124]

"Recently," he wrote Olive, "using our own sophisticated…microscopes, I have seen things with my own eyes that I know by training 'can't be true.' But they are." And he discovered that others had seen similar things, but had been laughed at and persecuted. "We need to bring together a small cadre of skilled scientists who can bridge the disciplines of medicine, chemistry, physics and biology." His real hope

---

123 Letter, Riordan to Olive Garvey, October 24, 1988, Office Files, CIHF Archives.
124 Interview, Dr. Hugh Riordan with Craig Miner, June 3, 1998.

was to announce on Olive W. Garvey's 100th birthday "that we have discovered how and why cancer develops, how to prevent it and how to treat it." It was a long shot, but pure Riordan. "Obviously, if my goal of achieving this 'impossible dream' is accomplished no other funding for The Center will ever be needed. I have long wondered what our true mission was. Now, I think I know."[125] And so the Garvey Center approached the last decade of the 20th century.

One more thing remained, however — the name. Olive had been insistent that it be changed. There must be a name, she said, by which CIHF "may be referred to. It is a puzzle to everybody including myself. I have to go through the initials before I can remember what its name is, and other people have even more trouble. When I want to mention it, I feel presumptuous reciting the whole title." Everything needed a title that was a kind of shorthand. "The banks call themselves The Fourth, The First.... The University is WSU." The Center could be called by initials, but "the general public is baffled by so many initials." She "wracked her brain" and came up with a suggested list.[126] Finally, early in 1990, she inquired why not just leave the "OWG" off the name and add "International?"[127] There were more than 300 donors by 1990 other than Olive and she thought some change was most appropriate. Therefore it was done. The new name, beginning in 1990, was "The Center for the Improvement of Human Functioning International, Inc," still a mouthful, but maybe more descriptive.[128]

The future was The Center's business, and it spent time regularly thinking about it. In October 1985, for example, shortly after moving into the Master Facility, the staff got together to imagine what the press would be saying about the CIHF in the year 2000 on its 25th anniversary. The collection of "Letters from the Future" revealed great hope and a wry sense of humor. Supposedly looking back from the future, the writers, now elderly, recalled those hard times in the late 1980s. "How

---

125 Letter, Riordan to Olive Garvey, October 24, 1988, Office Files, CIHF Archives.
126 Letter, Olive Garvey to Riordan, April 1, ibid.
127 Ibid, Jan. 28, 1990.
128 Media release, Feb. 9, 1990, History Scrapbook #3, CIHF Archives.

well I remember that tiny group of people who dared to face change and grow from it," one wrote. "No person could have seen what chance would entail." By the year 2000 war had been eliminated by discovering that "all our fears *were* in our heads." The Center had had a big role in eliminating fear from the world. Said another: "Remember in 1985 when our newly constructed Master Facility leaked like a sieve." But The Center had collected millions and fixed them all. In 1987 another projected that the American Medical Association had almost closed The Center down, but the World Health Organization intervened. The hypothetical backward glance continued: By 2000 The Center's international air shuttle system allowed people from all over the world to be at Dome #1 in an hour. In 1991 underground housing was built for those visitors on the "west side of the suspended transport system" (which used to be called a highway). The first Nobel Peace Prize for Research had been awarded to The Center in 1993. A second prize went to the African edible leaves project in 1994 which completely eliminated world hunger. The Nobel prize money was used by The Center to open a branch in Central Mexico, where a staff of 1,000 was nearly equal to the staff of the main facility in Wichita. The imagination continued to soar: "Health insurance companies were forced out of business by rising costs and eliminated in the year 1995." Meanwhile "people mainly flocked to us for help in slowing the aging process and exercise therapy." By the year 2000 many of The Center's doctors were former staff members from the bankrupt health insurance companies or leftovers from the American Medical Association, which was dissolved when the American Holistic Medical Association took over as the leading authority on health.[129]

It did not happen just that way, but it was not the last time the staff got together for some serious dreaming. At a minimum, it kept them healthier, they thought.

---

[129] "To the 25th Anniversary Committee, Oct. 15, 1985, History Scrapbook #2, ibid.

Chapter Seven
A New Era

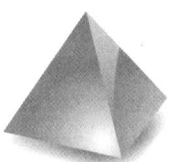

Early in the morning of May 4, 1993, Olive White Garvey, 99 years old, died at home with Dr. Riordan at her side. To say, as *Throwing a Rope* did, that she was "a great lady we treasured here at The Center," was the best that words could do.[1] Her birthday had always been a special event at the CIHF, and on what would have been her 100th birthday that July, The Center staff and friends celebrated for the first time in a long while without her, but in her honor.[2] "She could dominate without being domineering," said her son Willard. "No one would ever accuse her of trying to take charge of everything. They just gravitated to her." Bob Page added: "She was a true lady in a real sense of the word. Utterly without pretense…. She was the best business executive, male or female, I've ever been exposed to…. She had a great understanding of other people's problems. She had great intellectual curiosity. That's what kept her alive and alert for so long."

All of those qualities had helped The Center. Dr. Riordan remembered especially her wide reading and her ability to judge character. "She could look you in the eye and size you up. She was always so

---

1 *Rope*, May 10, 1993.
2 Ibid, July 19, 1993.

well-versed in anything she was dealing with that no one was going to be able to pull the wool over her eyes." Riordan said that Garvey knew more about nutrition than anyone with whom he had ever talked. Most important to him and to his enterprise, she was, as she once put it, "born with a contrary mind." The statement "it's always been done that way" was a red flag to her. "Shoot if you must this old gray head," she had written in one of her occasional poems, "but open up your mind, she said."3

The Center for the Healing Arts, with Dr. Hunninghake as Medical Director, was renamed the Olive W. Garvey Center for Healing Arts with Dr. Hunninghake as Director. And well it might be. Olive had provided a renewable research commitment for The Center she worked so hard for in life. $4.7 million was segregated in the Olive White Garvey Trust for the benefit of The Center, which would provide nearly $500,000 a year in support for the rest of time.4 "You might not know it," Riordan had written her in 1990, "but you provide me with a great deal of strength."5

Much of Riordan's recent correspondence with Garvey had concerned RECNAC. Most of the rest of it concerned the money The Center owed the Garvey Trust and had been unable to recover in the Messner litigation. As always, their relationship moved from the sublime, the visionary, to the practical, often in the space of a few sentences.

A few months after the Garvey funeral Riordan was interviewed by a health magazine called *Let's Live*. He was, the reporter said, "a large-framed man with a disarming sense of humor," and was "unexpectedly self-effacing." He explained that the odd shape of his head was due to genetic factors — his Irish, Russian, French, German and Mongolian blood — not to a difficult delivery at birth. Then the man, who by then could legitimately be called "one of the nation's top nutritionally

---

3 *Wichita Eagle*, May 5, 1993, History Scrapbook #3, CIHF Archives.
4 Letter, Robert Page to Hugh Riordan, October 20, 1993, Office Files, CIHF Archives.
5 Letter, Riordan to Olive Garvey, September 23, 1990, ibid.

oriented doctors" again explained his method and his goals. He and his staff of 42, he explained, treated ABNA patients of whom other physicians were happy to be rid. They had a 95% clearance rate for treating migraines. And patients not only felt better, they knew why. Riordan introduced them to the Mabee Library in Dome #2 on the first day. "That way," he noted, "the relationship is not just a smart doctor telling dumb patients what to do."

No doubt progress in alternative medicine would continue to be slow, and there would be battles still to fight, despite the establishment of considerable momentum in the last decade of the 20th century. He noted that it took those who knew that fresh fruits could cure scurvy about 200 years to prevail strongly enough to change the dietary practices of the British navy. Meanwhile over one million sailors died of the ailment, more than in all the battles of the era. The theory that blood circulated in the body was laughed at for many years. The stethoscope took 47 years to be accepted. The pattern was still present. "If what we are describing is (medically) acceptable, it's called a case study. If it's not acceptable, it's called 'anecdotal.'"[6]

No, time had not softened the attacks on alternative medicine that still came. The Proxmire bill of 1976 had limited the Food and Drug Administration to insuring that nutritional supplements met defined standards of purity and dosage. It passed after a public outcry when the FDA had tried to interfere with the public's right to buy these supplements.[7] But the agency still thought it should have more regulatory power in the health supplements field. Dr. David Kessler, head of the FDA, spoke in the standard vein when he told a congressional committee in 1993 that with the explosive growth of the health food and supplements industry "we are literally back at the turn of the century when snake-oil salesmen made claims for their products that could not be substantiated." But he had a special ax to grind and did recognize the interest.[8] Dr. Donald Davis responded to an editorial on

---

6 *Kansas Magazine*, (Fall, 1993), History Scrapbook #4, CIHF Archives.
7 *Rope*, December 9, 1991.
8 *Wichita Eagle*, August 12, 1993, ibid.

Kessler's statements in the local paper, characterizing it as "reckless." Davis wrote that, "Supplements are among the safest products Americans consume, far safer than aspirin, junk foods, coffee, alcohol, and tobacco."[9] The Center added in its newsletter that of 34 major pesticides used on lawns, 32 had not been tested for their long term effects on human beings. So why focus on vitamins?[10]

But amid the continued attacks, there was much evidence that more of the world was coming to Davis's perspective and to The Center's way of doing things. Sidney Harris, the syndicated columnist, wrote about medical "mavericks" in a 1991 column, comparing them to Gregor Mendel and the Wright brothers. The scientific enterprise, he commented, "has become increasingly bureaucratized, more specialized and heavily invested.... The maverick, obviously, does not nourish this self-serving system, and thus he is snubbed. The central problem in scientific discovery is that it is devilishly hard at first to tell a 'nut' from a 'genius.'" But "a society committed to the search for truth must give protection to, and set a high value upon, the independent and original mind, however angular, however socially unpleasant it may be; for it is upon such minds that the search for truth depends." There was scandal at the same time about the high overhead of many scientific labs, as much as 74%. The Center's overhead was never more than just over 20%. In the 1990s it was held to 15%. At Johns Hopkins, by contrast, it was 68%.[11] In the fall of 1993 there was a conference in Toronto sponsored by the *Journal of Otrhomolecular Medicine* and the Canadian Schizophrenia Foundation called "The Coming of Age of Nutritional Medicine." The presenters found it a situation "imbued with irony" that after years of ridicule alternative practitioners seemed on the verge of acceptance by the mainstream medical establishment. The largest hospitals and medical schools were confirming that "vitamin therapy is safe, inexpensive and effective in the treatment of many diseases."

---

9 Dr. Donald Davis to *Wichita Eagle*, September 1, 1993, ibid.
10 *Wichita Eagle,*, September 16, 1993, ibid.
11 *Rope*, January 9, 1991. Interview, Dr. Hugh Riordan with Craig Miner, October 22, 1998.

A New Era

Half of the attendees were physicians, and several were speaking about nutritional treatments for cancer.[12]

The popular interest in self-help and nutrition for health helped The Center locally, as did the building of a new northeast circumferential highway around Wichita. The construction caused access problems for a time, but when the freeway was completed in 1992, it not only made getting to The Center very convenient, but the view of it from the elevated roadway was spectacular, especially at night.[13] Local wag Bob Goetz in a 1994 column on the top 70 reasons why Wichita was a great place to live listed as #33: "That weird-looking holistic clinic on North Hillside that you can tell visitors is anything you want because no one really has the courage to go find out for sure what it is."[14]

The people who drove by might be reading Dean Ornish's latest diet book, in which he argued you could "Eat More, Weigh Less," by limiting calories from fat to 10% of one's diet. Nathan Pritikin had popularized something similar in the 1970s, but now low-fat diets (Scarsdale and Atkins were others) were a kind of cottage industry. Sodium became a culprit too. Ornish followed up with a second book on reversing heart disease through nutrition. Dr. Davis, The Center's consultant, was interviewed locally about these books. While he did not recommend such an extreme low-fat diet, he did agree that nutrition mattered, and was glad more were discovering it. In 1993, Mutual of Omaha insurance agreed to reimburse patients who participated in Ornish's diet-based disease prevention program.[15] Dr. Roger Williams when in his 90s still wrote about the benefits of nutrition, and the effect on aging, now with considerable credibility.[16]

The positive trend was clear in Wichita. The first *Taste of Health* cookbook, published by The Center's restaurant and including its tasty and

---

12 *Let's Live* (September., 1993), ibid.
13 *Rope*, July 2, 1990, February 3, 1992.
14 *Wichita Eagle*, November 21, 1994, History Scrapbook #4, CIHF Archives.
15 *Wichita Eagle*, Oct. 6, 1993, ibid.
16 Dr. Roger Williams, "What Improved Nutrition has Done for Me," *Positive Health*, (April/May, 1995), ibid.

healthy entrees, sold out almost immediately.[17] "Dreaded diet food," a local reporter said, could taste good.[18] In 1994 Madeline Coffman, a volunteer with a long background of idealistic work all over the world, joined The Center's volunteer staff with her husband Bob, a retired chemistry teacher who had expertise useful to the lab. She began teaching yoga at The Center, another element of Cornish's regimen for reducing heart disease.[19] "I'm a health nut," Coffman said. "I think the whole thing is to be healthy so you won't pick up diseases and need expensive treatments. God put us here to enjoy life. We like to be around young people and exposed to new ideas." The Coffmans were typical of The Center's volunteer force. "We don't have wealth to give," they said, "but what we have we can share and that's our time and our ability."[20] The Coffmans and others were examples of The Center's practicing what it preached about the continued usefulness of healthy people of an older age. In 1996, there were four octogenarians working or volunteering there, including prominently Nelda Reed, who never failed to greet visitors and wish them a nice day, and who had taken up modeling and ridden a motorcycle for the first time in her late seventies.[21]

Constantly, in fact, employees came from unexpected places. Dang Nguyen, for example, who became head of The Center's maintenance department, started work there in 1989 having arrived directly from Viet Nam with minimal knowledge of English. Dang had been a helicopter pilot in the South Vietnamese army, later a prisoner, and had tried escaping with the "boat people" several times before succeeding. He worked under cultural handicaps for the time, but The Center was just the kind of place to recognize potential and to provide opportunity.[22]

There were always good chances, too, for existing employees to change focus. Marsha McCray, for example, became a specialist in auricular therapy after extensive observation and training. Her first

---

17 *Rope*, June 11, 1990.
18 *Wichita Eagle*, March 4, 1994, History Scrapbook #4, CIHF Archives.
19 Clipping, January 22, 1994, in ibid.
20 *O.K. Times*, (November, 1994), ibid.
21 *Wichita Eagle*, November 6, 1996, ibid.
22 Interview, Laura Benson with Craig Miner, Sept. 10, 1999.

patient was Marge Page, the pioneer in so many things, but by the turn of the 21st century this variant of accupunture that worked on pain by using electrical impulses on parts of the ear was a very popular treatment. It was economical, and it was effective.[23]

And not only did people who had at first no expertise in a certain field gain it at The Center, but others who had so much expertise that they were skeptical of The Center's work got a chance to have their scientific minds convinced. Into the latter category falls James Jackson, PhD, who came to Wichita in 1983 to work at WSU and started working with The Center as its lab director in 1987. Jackson had worked for a lab that made a product called a "C stick," which The Center used in some of its tests. He was able to get them a supply of this product after it had gone out of production and subsequently started to work as a consultant at The Center and then as head of its laboratory.

Like so much else, the lab, when Jackson started working with it, was being cut in its funding from Garvey and forced to be more self-sufficient. The first year he was there it was subsidized at $55,000 a year, the second at $32,000, the third at nothing. It managed to make the transition and generate more income — $600,000 in 1998. According to Jackson, the lab did more with fewer staff members than any other lab of which he knew and served as a reference lab for tests in demand all over the country for research, but which for-profit labs could not afford to take the time to perform. Customers included the Mayo Clinic and Massachusetts General Hospital. Jackson's acquaintance with Chinese medicine, along with his experience at setting up laboratories in China, was also of help to The Center. Through him it attacted Dr. Xiao Long Meng, who became a key player in cancer research.

Jackson was a cynic at first about the value of nutrition. After a time, however, he was amazed that others could not see the sense of it. The body, after all, cannot make minerals, and all of them are essential. They must come through diet. The most common complaints of

---

23 Interview, Marsha McCray with Craig Miner, Sept. 10, 1999.

all patients are chronic fatigue, headache, joint and muscle pain. And these are precisely the symptoms of malnutrition.

Under Jackson's leadership the lab increased the number of tests it could perform by about 20%, without additional overhead, and at the end of the century was doing many, like parasitic and cytotoxic tests, that few labs in the country were equipped to do. Support from patients, who, after all, paid for every test, meant that it was able to maintain state-of-the art equipment.[24]

Over and over the cases were encouraging. There was success with carpal tunnel syndrome, almost a fad disorder of the 1990s it seemed, as office workers at computers were more and more affected. Many surgeries and/or rounds of cortisone injections were avoided by use of intravenous vitamin C and intramuscular vitamin B therapy.[25] There was success treating macular degeneration with zinc and selenium, and journal articles began to report that effectiveness.[26] Lead chelation continued. The Center got approval from USD 259 to do lead testing in the public schools, though funding was never forthcoming. The point was that there were probably 5,000 students in the Wichita schools who were not performing as well as they could due to lead in their systems.[27] A hyperbaric oxygen unit was installed at The Center and used for osteomyletis, peripheral vascular disease, and many other ailments.[28] That came about because years before Riordan had referred a patient with circulatory problems in his legs to the only hospital that had one, requesting that he be given 12 one hour hyperbaric treatments, but after 3 half hour ones they amputated his leg without calling Riordan back. He vowed then to get his own unit.[29] At Center-sponsored health fairs, people had their vitamin C, cholesterol, zinc, lead and vitamin E levels checked, getting the results for some of the tests in an hour. "And Dr. Hugh had the pleasure

---

24 Interview, Dr. James Jackson with Craig Miner, Sept. 10, 1999.
25 *Rope*, June 18, 1990.
26 Ibid, May 31, 1988.
27 Ibid, June 3, 1991.
28 Ibid, Aug. 24, 1992.
29 Interview, Dr. Hugh Riordan with Craig Miner, October 22, 1998.

of giving hugs to more than 750 people."[30] And the stand bys, like migraines, continued to have high success rates. One man wrote in 1993 that his wife had had migraines for 20 years. She had to quit work, miss some of the children's activities, and spend hours in the dark. She consulted with many neurologists, took injections that cost $60 a day and had high bills for visits to doctors. The couple knew of The Center, but knew also that insurance would not pay for it. But finally they went anyway. Within 30 days, the woman was taking less medication, spending less, and getting better. She ended up spending six cents a day for vitamin C, and their daughter, formerly on heavy antibiotics, was helped also.[31] There were applications of vitamin C to help dental bleeding.[32] Neil Riordan, Dr. Hugh Riordan's son, discovered at The Center's lab in 1994 a way of identifying a pesky parasite, *Dientamoeba Fragilis*, which caused patients digestive problems.[33] The Center could even ward off mosquitoes with vitamin B1 or prevent motion sickness with ginger.[34]

The "Bright Spot for Health" fair in June 1993 attracted 1,500 people despite torrential rains. There were free lectures, food, and games for children as well as the laboratory tests. It brought many people to The Center campus who had not been to the facility before. The event involved all staff and a tremendous turnout of volunteers also. There was a test putting a drop on the tongue which indicated by color the ability of the system to assimilate Vitamin C. There were grip tests, lung capacity tests, and many others different than the standard blood pressure and weight estimates one got at the standard physical. It was a chance too to inform a broader public about The Center's program.[35]

Of course, there were the cancer cases. Even when the cancer remained and the patient died, the families thanked The Center for

---

30 *Rope*, June 21, 1993.
31 Ibid, August 30, 1993.
32 Ibid, Oct. 24, 1994.
33 Ibid, November 7, 1994. *Wichita Eagle*, November 11, 1994, History Scrapbook #4, CIHF Archives.
34 *Wichita Eagle*, June 2, 1994, History Scrapbook #4, CIHF Archives.
35 Interview, Laura Benson and Marilyn Landreth with Craig Miner, Aug. 27, 1999.

increasing the quality of life remaining to their loved ones. One MD wrote in 1997 thanking The Center for helping his 83-year-old father who had come there with a diagnosis of 30-60 days left to live. He was bed-ridden, had severe pain and a defeated attitude. The son heard a lecture by Riordan on vitamin C, began treating his father with it, was able to cut his pain medication by 50%, and his color and attitude increased remarkably. Before he died he was even able to get out of bed and meet his friends for lunch.[36]

Many case summaries were equally as moving. In 1986, The Center began treatment of an autistic four-year-old. His mother had wondered "if there were alternatives to simply 'managing' symptoms," and so came to the domes on North Hillside. He was found to have low levels of several nutrients, especially zinc. The Center worked also to improve his amino acid metabolism, candida levels, tolerance to food, and overall digestive function. "Gradually," his mother wrote, "we learned what had a negative effect on his system and what didn't." A single exposure to dairy products, for example, resulted in loss of eye contact for 24 hours. Exposure to gluten-containing grains resulted in reduced motor control. Step by step he was helped. By 1992 the boy was an enthusiastic and successful fourth grader, a Webelo scout, a soccer player, and a martial arts specialist. "The Center," his mother wrote then, "has strengthened our family's belief in the power of everyday individuals and informed, committed groups to effect positive, meaningful change. Without question, it has given us a new sense of 'the possible.'"[37]

The files at The Center's 20th anniversary in 1995 were thick with testimonials: "Coming to The Center has made me aware of my body and that I am in charge of my own wellness." "Let me express my gratitude for the pioneer spirit that still exists here in Wichita, where new, nonstandard approaches can flourish if they are worthwhile." "The Center was a life saver for Billy. Before we came to The Center, the doctors were saying we should have our little child committed. Coming to The Center for food sensitivity and other testing has influenced his life positively in

---

36 *Rope,* November 17, 1997.
37 Ibid, October 2, 1996.

every way…. Billy went on to college and became a teacher and a coach. He married a lovely woman this year." "When I came to The Center, I had to have my wife put on my socks, I was so stiff from my arthritis. Because of the help I received at The Center, I am completely pain and symptom free today." "Before coming to The Center I had a life of constant pain. The Center brought me back to the world of joy and life — physically, mentally and spiritually. You don't know how dark your inner world becomes with constant pain." "After my cancer treatment, they just sent me home and said I was cured without doing anything to help me fix my body from the damage done by the treatment. I came to The Center to do just that, to change my internal environment for the better." "At 71 and 2/3 years of age, I feel more physically empowered and in better health than I did when I was 20 years younger. The Center is one of the biggest reasons for my well being." "When I started with Dr. Riordan, I had been told I needed my right knee and left hip replaced, arthritis in my upper and lower extremities, cataracts in both eyes and many other problems. Today I am approaching 79 years young, and work 33 hours a week, have all my original joints without arthritis and see clearly without having cataract surgery. Isn't that good?"[38]

And that kind of response continued. A request for personal histories in 1997, anticipating the 25th anniversary, led to a flurry of them: "Walking through the doors at The Center, each and every time, gave us the feeling of being wrapped in hope, love and peace. My husband lost his life to cancer but not the battle. Thanks to prayers and the treatment at The Center he died with no pain."[39] "After going from one doctor to another for 26 years and constantly being prescribed Lomotel and Valium, Dr. Ron Hunninghake diagnosed my illness and saved my life."[40] "Usually I dread going to the doctor. However, I now actually look forward to driving 2 1/2 hours to see you all. When I came here, I had absolutely no hope that I would *ever* feel well again."[41] "The

---

38 20th Anniversary souvenir flyer, 1995, History Scrapbook #4, CIHF Archives.
39 Carol Dale to Riordan, November 25, 1997, Office Files, CIHF Archives.
40 Ruby Harrington, November 11, 1997, ibid.
41 Bliss Burnham to Riordan, November 14, 1997, ibid.

Center has been helpful. They give you the feeling that your slightest complaint is important & they want you to feel better. The regular doctors feel that your slightest complaint is not life threatening so why worry about it."[42] "Your work is transformational work, and it is sacred work.... Hugh Riordan will be remembered as a 20th century giant of the future and as a miracle worker."[43] "The DOCTOR was really IN."[44] While people are always appreciative of good medical care in their times of crisis, it is unlikely many doctors' offices have such a personal collection.

The only "problem" with these regular case successes was that they were ordinary ailments of ordinary people. One of The Center's supporters wrote in 1990 that "the trouble with you folks at The Center is that you don't do anything that grabs me in the gut." The staff thought it could live with that. In a way the lack of drama was part of the mission of promoting wellness rather than intervening in sickness. "Chasing fire engines and seeing a fire is more exciting than preventing fires. Preventing birth defects is boring compared to the excitement of a newborn intensive care unit and the gut-wrenching appearance of severely deformed infants. Preventing cancer seems less important than treating those afflicted with the disease." And, of course, it was much more difficult to document and to sell a disaster avoided than one softened.[45] Still, as the *Rope* put it in 1996: "Compared to the hundreds of millions of dollars poured into this year's political campaigns or the weekly take of casinos in Las Vegas, our needs are very small."[46]

RECNAC was a major focus, and it did provide a higher profile and more drama. Cancer was just the kind of chronic, metabolic disease in which The Center specialized, but because it was so dangerous and so often terminal, and because the ordinary treatments were so drastic, there was great interest in prevention and alternative treatment.

---

42 Jo Berchtold to Riordan, November 12, 1997, ibid.
43 Bill Manahan, M.D. to Riordan, November 3, 1997, ibid.
44 Barbara Peterson to Riordan, October 29, 1997, ibid.
45 *Rope*, July 22, 1990.
46 Ibid, November 7, 1996.

A New Era

The Center had had patients with cancer for a long time. Zelma Barackman, for instance, had a lump in her breast in 1985, which seemed to get bigger and was found to be cancerous. She had it surgically removed, but, as a registered nurse, she knew that three needle biopsies could have leaked cancer cells into her body, and there was a possibility that the cancer was not totally removed. She also stated that she had the care of three elderly people and she just did not have time to go through the sickness connected with the recommended radiation and chemotherapy. Instead she asked for a referral to the CIHF "That absolutely blew their [the doctors'] minds," she remembered.[47]

Barackman, however, was a reader. She had read an article in *Psychology Today* about cancer's being a kind of "death wish," which could be reversed by visual imagery. At her first meeting with Dr. Riordan, she said she did not want chemotherapy. He said, "Then don't do it." She couldn't believe it, but was gratified. She read Norman Cousins's book *Anatomy of an Illness* and began thinking that "what the mind sees, the body believes. We create our own reality. We can be much in charge." It was a time of great stress in her family, and she reasoned she had had an unconscious wish to be ill. As a nurse trained in the 1940s, she did not like to talk back to doctors, but this time she did. "I'm not afraid of death," she said. "I just didn't want to die slowly. I wanted to live hard and die fast. I didn't want to be sick. I wanted a quality of life, not a quantity." She put her husband's mother in a nursing home, got call waiting, and began treatment at The Center.[48] Ten healthy years later, she was convinced she had made the right choice. When people asked her how she was doing, she would respond: "I don't know, how do I look?"

Part of what Barackman did at The Center was to learn to use visual imaging. She had the feeling cancer cells were all over her body, and was asked to come up with an image for getting rid of them. She remembered a time when her husband and she were in Silverton, Colorado watching a sheepherder bring in sheep. She visualized a corral in her body and

---

47 clipping, July 15, 1995, History Scrapbook #4, CIHF Archives. Interview, Marilyn Landreth with Craig Miner, Aug. 27, 1999.
48 "I Chose Life," *Hutchinson News*, March 30, 1997, ibid.

sent out little black and white dogs to gather cancer cells and bring them into that corral and dispose of them "however was natural." Barackman talked to many other cancer patients about her positive experience.[49]

Opal Williams's husband developed cancer of the kidney in 1985, and it spread into his lung and liver, showing up in six spots. The recommendation was chemotherapy, with a 15-20% chance of recovery. They came to see Dr. Riordan. "He promised us nothing," but there had been some reports of vitamin C being effective, and her husband took that for six weeks. He died of a heart attack 12 years later with no evidence of cancer. Mrs. Williams at 88 wrote Riordan to thank him "for giving me my husband for 12 years."[50]

Richard Lewis recalled the first contact with another cancer patient. During the ABNA project he was working at the desk one Friday afternoon in October when a "tall, rather imposing woman" came in and said she wanted to be in the program. Lewis told her there were no openings until January of next year. Her response was to lean over the counter and say: "I don't have time to wait, I was just told that I have cancer and will be dead before Christmas." That got Lewis's attention. There was a cancellation the next Monday, The Center forwent the usual two weeks of paperwork and started treatments immediately. The patient was a Roman Catholic nun. She saw that Christmas and three more before cancer took her, and in that time established an holistic retreat center at Great Bend, Kansas, modeled after the CIHF.[51]

"We are looking at cancer," said Riordan in his 1993 interview, "as an adaptive mechanism. The body is trying to adapt to something and what it is adapting to is inadequate nutrients in the presence of other adequate nutrients. Our research philosophy is to observe nature and then to model it in the laboratory, rather than to come up with our own solution and force it on nature." It had been known for decades that vitamin A and Beta Carotene were nutrients that helped prevent and could even reverse cancer by eliminating free radicals created by

---

49 Clipping, July 15, 1995, History Scrapbook #4, CIHF Archives.
50 Opal Williams to Riordan, October 30, 1997, Office Files, CHIF archives.
51 Richard Lewis, "Thoughts on The Center," 1997, ibid.

oxidization. The Center expanded on that research and was studying at that moment a slime mold called physarum that grew on forest trees. It was a model for cancer in that it grew one way until it ran out of nutrients, then sent up a stalk, almost like a polyp in the colon. That stalk grew and then blew -- it metastasized and spread from one area to another in search of food. Maybe human cancers did that. Or maybe a copy machine was a better analogy, where the DNA, the boss, told the RNA, the secretary, to make copies on white paper. But if the secretary brought back copies on yellow paper, all the DNA knew was that it did not get what it wanted, so sent her back for more. And the unwanted copies caused havoc. Riordan used a variety of analogies for a reporter or to anyone, including especially cancer patients.[52]

The Center did raise money for RECNAC, not the $20 million endowment it wanted, but about $1.4 million the first year.[53] There were new sources, including now foundations. The West Trust, for example, contributed $20,600 in 1991, and the Wallace Genetic Foundation of New York City gave $30,000.[54] Early in 1990, a list of "research premises" was published: 1) that cancer is the manifestation of a most fundamental process basic to life, 2) that cancer is 100% genetic and 100% epigenetic, 3) that cancer is a systemic phenomenon, 4) that cancer is an adaptive process rather than an invader, 5) that cancer development and suppression involves multiple intercommunication activities, 6) that cancer develops in response to an interruption of effective cellular micro environments which are controlled by fill-hold-release sequences at the cellular and sub cellular levels, 7) that cancer develops over a prolonged period of time, 8) that cancer development is pleomorphic involving several stages which do not resemble each other, 9) that the keys to understanding the development of cancer will be found through concurrent modeling and intensely observing the interplay between multiple biologic systems, 10) that to understand the development of cancer, The Center needed to bring together sci-

---

52 *Kansas Magazine*, (Fall, 1993), History Scrapbook #4, CIHF Archives.
53 *Rope*, Februrary 12, 1990.
54 Ibid, March 4, 1991.

entists in the disciplines of biophysics, chronobiology, developmental biology, electromagnetic spectral engineering, experimental pathology, genetic biochemistry, microbiology, molecular biology, photobiology, and radiation physics.[55]

In connection with RECNAC, The Center developed the MIMIC lab, a $450,000 facility made possible by a grant from the Mabee Foundation, whose design was fundamental to the evolving philosophy.[56] It was the first lab in the world where the multiple factors of light, temperature and electromagnetic fields were controlled so that cells could be studied in conditions resembling living tissue. A reporter was entertained at a 1993 visit:

> After stepping on two sets of sticky mats, one passes through the air lock entrance into the general laboratory space, lighted only with subdued ultraviolet. There is an awareness that one has entered a different type of environment. And it is. After a short while, one's eyes adjust to the low level of light and everything becomes clearly visible. The interior is white. The walls, the ceiling, the cabinetry, and all surfaces are white to better reflect the very low level of light. Large blackboard-like writing surfaces are on the walls of the outer laboratory, but they are white, written on with colors that fluoresce under the ultraviolet light.

The visitor was told this was a place where history would be made. Certainly it was a state of the art lab for study at the cellular level and a far cry from that first 1975 Center lab on East Douglas.[57]

Developments came quickly and were shared. Researchers at the National Cancer Institute had written as early as 1969 that the future of effective chemotherapy was not in toxic compounds, but non-toxic

---

55 Ibid.
56 *Wichita Eagle*, July 15, 1992, History Scrapbook #4, CIHF Archives.
57 *Rope*, January 18, 1993.

A New Era

ones. That was The Center's direction. In 1993 it published a second set of research assumptions: 1) that normal cells are aerobic; cancer cells are partial anaerobes and cannot survive in an oxygen rich environment ; 2) in nature the primary reason cells change their behavior is that they run out of essential nutrients; cancer cells are cells that have changed their behavior; 3) The Center's research showed that specific nutrients were effective not only in reducing the growth of some cancer cells but in selectively killing them.[58]

In 1994 came another provocative list including two completely new items: 1) The Center did not treat cancer; it treated the individual who happened to have cancer, 2) it asked "why does it make sense to the body to be producing cancer?"[59] It was also working on a way to diagnose cancer without biopsies, as the biopsy testing method was thought to spread the disease.[60] By then RECNAC had developed consulting relationships with people all over the country, and had many breakthroughs at various levels. It had developed a new reliable lab method for determining the number of live and dead cells in a cultured system, it had increased the speed of scanning for anti-tumor activity by 60 fold, it had developed a new reliable enzymatic-based method for differentiating between normal and tumor cells, it had patented a spin-off technique to identify intestinal parasites using fluorescing dyes and ultraviolet microscopy, it had determined that in cell culture vitamin C was preferentially cytotoxic to 11 different types of cancers, it had determined in cell cultures the optimal exposure time for vitamin C to yield its maximum result among cancer cells, it had used infrared techniques to determine specific frequencies which were selectively absorbed by tumor cells, and it was using new specially designed incubators to determine that some tumor cells were profoundly affected by minimal changes in temperature.[61] There were publications arising from that research, including one entitled "Improved Microplate

---

58 Ibid, January 25, 1993.
59 Ibid, Feburary 7, 1994.
60 *Wichita Eagle*, February 12, 1994.
61 *Rope*, February 7, 1994.

Fluormeter Counting of Viable Tumor and Normal Cells," published in *Anti-Cancer Research*. Patents also were forthcoming. The Center instituted a relationship with the Beijing Tumor Institute in China to perform animal studies and moved to establish relationships with university medical school oncology departments for larger scale testing. Overhead expenses stayed at 15%, and The Center noted that it "looked upon with increasing satisfaction the accelerating awareness among medical researchers that certain nutrient related compounds may be key factors in the prevention and non-toxic treatment of cancer." Some cancer patients diagnosed as terminal and treated by The Center had lived nine years, and their continued quality of life was monitored. [62]

Patients volunteered to try new techniques. Several with pancreatic cancer, which usually had a very short survival time, had been helped by high dose vitamin C. Riordan had tried vitamin C on pancreatic cancer for the first time in 1980. The patient died, but 18 months after the predicted date. In 1983 he had tried a higher dose with another man. "When he came, I didn't think he'd last a week." The man traveled and pursued other interests. His tumor disappeared for a time, but eventually reappeared and he died, but he had a year of quality life and never required hospitalization.[63] Now, in the mid-1990s, The Center sought out people who had cancer of the head of the pancreas and who had had surgery, but not chemotherapy and were free of liver metastases. For those people The Center would give one year of therapy, longer than the normal life expectancy, at no charge.[64]

On February 10, 2000, The Center announced the results of its RECNAC project, as promised. It had demonstrated that vitamin C is toxic to tumor cells at concentrations that are achievable with high dose intravenous infusions. It further showed that when vitamin C is combined with lipoic acid, the dose required for tumor-cell killing decreases. It demonstrated that vitamin C can be administered intra-

---

62 Press release, February 9, 1995, History Scrapbook #4, CIHF Archives.
63 *Wichita Eagle*, February 11, 1995.
64 *Rope*, Feburary 9, 1995.

venously at sustained doses of at least 50g/day for 8 weeks without causing renal complications or significant alterations in blood counts or chemistry profiles. It obtained evidence that vitamin C supplementation improves some parameters of immune cell functioning, and it had improved the condition of several cancer patients through the use of intravenous vitamin C, or a combination of intravenous vitamin C with other antioxidants and immune stimulating agents. The project also had developed and tested a non-toxic extract from a locally-grown plant which was capable of halting new blood vessel growth and inhibiting tumor growth. It developed an immune stimulant from bacterial culture that exhibited significant anti-tumor activity. The lab gained the ability to grow dendritic cells and train them with tumor antigens obtained from the patient or produced cheaply in the lab. These could be infused into patients to boost tumor-specific immune responses. It developed a method by which a patient's white blood cells could be used to produce an autologous cytokine cocktail and developed a protocol for administering this cocktail as a biological response modifier for cancer patients. Aiden, Inc., was formed, with Neil Riordan as president, to market some of the products coming from RECNAC research. It was not the end of cancer, but it was a strong list for the project.[65]

Riordan quoted Lewis Thomas that "trying to be useful and failing at it is the major source of discontent, driving some of us crazy." The thing that had been driving Riordan crazy was a "lurking fascination" over the question of whether standard research techniques were interfering with understanding of physiological processes. RECNAC was a chance to study that and a dread disease at the same time.[66]

There were many examples of the project's maintaining state of the art status. In 1996, it installed a special enclosure (a Faraday Cage) entirely free of electronic interference. Though one could see out of it through a meshwork, a radio would not receive inside.[67] In 1998, The Center for the Improvement of Human Functioning was selected

---

65 RECNAC report, Feb, 10, 2000, CIHF Archives.
66 Riordan statement, n.d., c. 1991, History Scrapbook #3, CIHF Archives.
67 *Rope*, February 20, 1996.

along with the Sloan Kettering Institute, St. Luke's Hospital, the Pacific Northwest Hospital, and the MD Anderson Hospital to test Dr. Gerald Murphy's dendritic cell therapy treatment for cancer. By far the smallest institution on the list, The Center, thanks to RECNAC, nevertheless had the sophisticated lab, the cancer experience, and the skilled staff the project required. Because of the need for cooperation with a local hospital which did not occur, that project did not go forward as planned.[68]

All the while, The Center, as always, spoke not only to the professionals, but to the public. And it spoke to them not only of life-threatening disease already contracted, but of chronic ailments not yet transformed from annoyance to threat. It hoped, too, that there would be some ills that a new generation could entirely avoid, never having to complain of any symptom at all.

The international conferences continued. The year 2000 marked the 15th. But the *Health Hunter* newsletter, better than any surviving record, documents The Center's month by month stance in the 1990s going out to 1,100 people. It grew in size and in quality. Richard Lewis remembered that at first it was difficult to find articles in the medical or popular press for reporting in *Hunter*, but by the 1990s that had all changed.[69] Not only was there plenty to report about from the broad world of alternative medicine, but more and more from the activities of The Center itself.

Donald Davis surprised in the January 1990 issue by informing readers that we ate 600 pounds of food a year, and that if our appetite control were off even 5% we would gain or lose 30 pounds a year. But it could be fooled by empty calories. Maybe not everyone was ready to substitute a slice of whole grain bread for a cookie. But, instead of eating three chocolate sandwich cookies, perhaps one could eat three fig bar cookies and save 4 grams of fat and 36 calories. Instead of a glazed donut, why not try a slice of angel food cake and save 110 calories, 13 grams of fat and 21 milligrams of cholesterol. Step by step, things

---

68 Interview, Neil Riordan with Craig Miner, April 16, 1998.
69 Interview, Richard Lewis with Craig Miner, June 3, 1998.

would change. Visitors to the CIHF could stop and check the computer at the entrance for the "nutricircle" analysis of any food or any meal free of charge. Similar-seeming ones can be vastly different, and "dismembered foods are obviously palatable -- too palatable." Davis, in a way typical of *Hunter's* practical editorials suggested: "First change *what* you eat, and let the *how much* take care of itself." Don't skip meals, don't use artificial sweeteners, eat only when you are hungry and slowly, and avoid eating large meals late in the day. "Don't just treat your taste buds," went a tip from the *Taste of Health* restaurant in the same issue. "Treat your whole body."[70]

Dr. Tinterow, who died in 1993 just before Olive Garvey, lived actively right up to the end, as The Center recommended. In February 1990 he contributed an article called "The Trend Toward Self-Responsibility." People who ate whole grain bread and preferred bottled water to mixed drinks, he said, were no longer in the 1990s thought of as "health nuts." A University of Chicago study showed that self-caring persons spent 26% less on hospital bills and 19% less on doctors than others. Between 1977 and 1981, just as The Center was beginning, sales of health related books nationwide went up 1100%. Tinterow thought that "when medical historians look back at the last quarter of the 20th century, they will see it as a period in which we moved from an old health care system built around the doctor, the hospital, and the clinic to a new health care system built around the individual, the family, and the home."[71]

There followed all sorts of specific advice: "Is Your Thyroid OK?," "Characteristics of Exceptional Patients," "Credibility," "Ever Consider a Walking Vacation?," "Dybosis: The Sick Gut Connection," "Human Intestinal Parasites," "Depression: Is There a Biological Base?," "Carpal Tunnel Syndrome (CTS): The Center's Approach," "Eating to Reduce Stress," "Cholesterol, Fat and Heart Disease: A Scientific Boondoggle?," "Healing Your Irritable Bowel," "Violence and Biochemistry," "I've Never Met a Bean I Didn't Like," "DHEA."

---

70 *Health Hunter*, vol. 4, no. 1 (January, 1990).
71 Ibid, vol. 4, no. 2 (February, 1990).

The same variety of subjects contained in the newsletter, and the same sort of compelling titles, filled the room at the luncheon lectures. People could eat a *Taste of Health* meal, hear a perfectly organized speech, for which they received a detailed outline, and, if they wished, purchase a video or audio cassette of the whole thing afterwards. The system had become very sophisticated. The banners on the driveway at the 25th anniversary would read "25 years helping people from 50 states and 33 foreign countries." It announced a health fair for school children in Kansas, called "Health Is," with prizes, as part of its ongoing program to help a new generation to a new kind of future.

Thomas Edison once wrote that : "The doctor of the future will give no medicine, but will interest his patients in the care of the human frame, in diet and in the cause and prevention of disease." William Osler had said something similar: "It is more important to know what sort of person has a disease than to know the sort of disease a person has." By the mid-1990s, it almost seemed that the day of change in medicine so long predicted had come. At a meeting of cardiologists in 1996, 70% said they took vitamin E regularly though no large studies proved it had an effect on heart disease. The National Institutes of Health had, by that time, established an Office of Alternative Medicine. There was more vitamin C in medicine cabinets than aspirin. [72] In 1998, the American Medical Association printed the news that B vitamins are useful and might even prevent heart attacks, something the CIHF had been teaching for decades.[73]

By the late 1990s, the trend was clear. The AMA *Journal* in 1998 published an entire issue devoted to alternative medicine, its lead article entitled "Alternative Medicine -- Learning from the Past, Examining the Present, Advancing to the Future." 40% of patients by that time were seeking non-standard aid for chronic disease problems, thanks partly to a "declining faith that scientific breakthroughs will have relevance for the personal treatment of disease." 60% of medical schools included some training in alternative medicine, and the

---

72 Ibid, vol. 10, no. 1 (January, 1996).
73 *Rope*, February 9, 1998.

National Institutes of Health budgeted $50 million a year to its study. "Alternative medicine is here to stay," wrote the *Journal*. "It is no longer an option to ignore it or treat it as something outside the normal process of science and medicine. The challenge is to move forward carefully, using both reason and wisdom, as we attempt to separate the pearls from the mud."[74] Denham Harman, MD, the father of the free radical theory of aging, found suddenly that the ideas he had been developing since 1945 attracted considerable publicity.[75] Also prominent was Judah Folkman, who for years had worked on a theory of cancer that shrank tumors by cutting off their blood supply rather than attacking them with toxic chemicals.[76] Immunologists had always sought what alternative medicine would call an orthomolecular solution to that disease, one that used the body's own resources for a cure. The University of Kansas Medical School established a division of Alternative Medicine, causing one local physician with whom Riordan spoke about it to say the news "made him want to vomit."[77] The *Wichita Eagle* contained headlines such as "Big Dose of B Vitamins May Cut Heart Risk," "Eat Your Way to a Cancer-Free Life, Study Stays," or "Sunlight Cuts Breast Cancer Risk," and these were not reporting on Alternative Medicine, but on standard medical studies.[78] An insurance broker attending one of Dr. Ron's luncheon lectures on the state of alternative medicine in 1999 inquired how she might work with The Center "to cover some of these therapies and services." Times had changed on that front also.[79]

Those developments pleased Dr. Hugh Riordan very much. He was characterized in an article entitled "Men You Should Know" in *Wichita Women* magazine in 1994 as "stress free, calm and confident, putting

---

74 Wayne Jonas, M.D., "Alternative Medicine -- Learning from the Past, Examining the Present, Advancing to the Future," *Journal of the American Medical Association* (November 11, 1998), pp. 1616-17.
75 "Father of the Free Radical Theory of Aging Looks Ahead," *Nutrition Science News*, vol. 3, No. 7 (July, 1998), pp. 344-48.
76 *Science* (May 15, 1998), p. 997.
77 Interview, Dr. Hugh Riordan with Craig Miner, October 22, 1998.
78 *Wichita Eagle*, October 1, November 4, November 20, 1997.
79 Lunch lecture evaluation, Aug. 24, 1999, CIHF Archives.

others around him at ease."[80] Swimming upstream against criticism, he had treated by 1995 over 11,000 patients at the CIHF from 26 countries and every state.[81] He had the testimonial letters and the personal scars to prove it.

As the millennium and the 25th anniversary of The Center approached he remained hardworking, calm, but outspoken. Certainly he was not satisfied, and saw the crusade and The Center going on well beyond his own demise. He was confident that The Center would be able to demonstrate in a significant number of people that it could deal with cancer with methods not damaging to human cells, and it would show that even if some of the testing had to be done abroad. As it was, the government could be a barrier, when, according to Riordan, it "should be paying for natural things that will be inexpensive and effective and don't have toxic side effects on normal cells."

His great pride was that The Center looked at peoples' entire life history rather than just at a last, or acute stage. And he was proud about involving the patient and changing the relationship between doctor and patient. He had a dream of teaching medical school on cable TV so everyone would be a better consumer. "It is quite amazing, from my standpoint, what people are told," and, more, what they would believe. But doctors had no time. "If you're down to a couple of minutes per patient, there is no choice but to blow them off." He also thought again about having sufficient funds to never again have to charge people at the time of service, but, as with the ABNA project, just to look to them for contributions as they were thankful for the help they had received. The Center continued to honor people who had been with it for more than 20 years, rather than getting rid of them as seemed true of some organizations.

The staff was doing what their education might have indicated, and that was the way Riordan liked it. There were many on the staff who had been there a decade or two and always understood that they had a job description plus whatever needed to be done. "People kind of fit in or don't fit in over time." And they pulled together very well.

---

80 *Wichita Women* (March, 1994), History Scrapbook #4, CIHF Archives.
81 Souvenir flyer for 20th anniversary, 1995, ibid.

Riordan was "not a thinker, I'm a perceiver." And he was happy with that — with being "a generalist in a kind of specialist's sort of way." He could see the point in the old saw about knowing more and more about less and less until we knew everything about nothing. "Learning," he said, "is just seeing what is here and what is over there. It's been a wonderful thing to observe and record for humankind whatever is working. It's been a lot of fun."

Had it mattered? Of course, and especially it had mattered to Wichita, a fact that would suit loyal native Olive Garvey, or Bob Page, who said that he lived in Wichita because it was as far as he could get simultaneously from New York and Los Angeles. Dr. Riordan had taken a risk and combined science with entrepreneurship to build a small opportunity and an almost chance meeting into a significant institution. The Center by the year 2000 had managed successfully the transition from heavy dependence upon a single benefactor to a broad base of support, a feat almost as rare as holding together a family business through a change of generations. The Center prepared for the change, educated all its staff about cost and income, and, as Laura Benson put it, when 1994 came "we were really all right. We continued to be all right." [82] The Center marketed well. It had levels of service for anyone, from the Mabee Library, which was free, to the luncheon lectures and the *Health Hunter* organization, which were very inexpensive, to levels of medical care ranging from the "Call the Doctor" program, to a "Beat the Odds" test.[83]

Riordan's daughter Renee commented that there were no Mercedes in the staff parking lot at The Center, but the staff was as close and motivated as it had been from the beginning, and people found not only health there, but peace and contentment.[84] The Center was not just a company with a product but a caring group with a mission: to create an epidemic of health. As Riordan put it in 1998: "There is such a change in medicine that I don't think you can go back."[85]

---

82 Interview, Laura Benson with Craig Miner, June 10, 1998.
83 Interview, Dr. Hugh Riordan with Craig Miner, October 22, 1998.
84 Interview, Renee Olmstead with Craig Miner, November 30, 1998.
85 Interview, Dr. Hugh Riordan with Craig Miner., June 10, 1998.

Epilogue

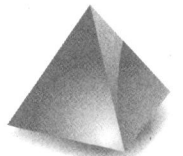

My husband, Hugh Riordan, was known for his work ethic, often spending 16 hours a day at his beloved Center for the Improvement of Human Functioning. On a cold, icy morning of Friday, January 7, 2005, Dr. Riordan was at work in his Clinic office. Shortly before noon, he wrote what would later be discovered to be his final thoughts — completing the last volume of his *Medical Mavericks* trilogy of great physicians. Minutes later he returned to his desk and collapsed. He died with his boots on — literally, as it was a snowy day — which is how he wanted it to be. It was fitting that he died doing what he loved and where he loved to be.

I wrestled mightily with the decision of whether to publish this manuscript. I questioned whether this was something that Hugh would want me to do. The fact that he himself did not publish it during his lifetime demonstrates his deep ambivalence about Craig Miner's account, which had been commissioned for The Center's 25th anniversary. Despite Hugh's genius, or maybe because of it, it was difficult for him to see himself in the third person. That is what Craig's account is — not a hagiography but rather a factual telling of the fascinating story of how two innovative people — Hugh and his patron Olive Garvey — in a Midwestern city during the late 20th Century went about their ambitious goal of transforming health care.

Among Hugh's "save" boxes, I found more unpublished versions of his life story (along with, believe it or not, a swatch of his white beard) written by different authors. One is by Marilyn Landreth, an early Center staff member. It's a fine piece of work and if the reader is into more information about Hugh I advise you to contact Marilyn Landreth at (marilake@cox.net) for a copy. I also found a detailed description and list of contents for a future book about Hugh that was drawn up by his good friend, the writer and artist Patric Rowley, but never came to being.

A third unfinished book I found was an autobiography by Hugh himself that included detailed descriptions of clinical cases. This was in response to colleagues asking for specific clinical information on various medical conditions and treatments. Sadly, it was never published. Given the aborted attempts to put his story into print, I proposed to Susan Miner, Craig's wife, that his manuscript be published, and she readily agreed that it would be a fitting tribute to both of our husbands.

I met Hugh in 1955 at a psychiatric facility in Madison, Wisconsin, where we both worked. I was a nurse and he a lab tech paying his way through Medical School. It was pretty much "love at first sight." I was dating someone else but he moved right into my life and we married.

Despite his heavy work schedule, Hugh supported me in my professional interests — mainly nursing. He encouraged me to go back to school to earn a doctorate and to teach nursing at the Wichita State University, which I did for 23 years. Aside from the many hours he spent at The Center he also joined me in working for La Leche League and serving on their International Board of Directors.

Our six children (4 sons, 2 daughters) had an interesting childhood. Hugh was as innovative a parent as he was a physician. For example, while other parents installed swing sets and slides in their backyards, Hugh dumped a truckful of dirt onto our little patch. The kids played on that little hill, tunneling through it and re-sculpting as their imaginations demanded. A unique dresser, to the delight of the neighbors, Hugh, shirtless, wore shorts and cowboy boots when working at home, even if the temperature was below freezing.

Hugh was, yes, a character. But he also had extraordinary strength of character. He had an unparalleled sense of fairness. He was a loving and dedicated father. And he strove to find the joy in everyday life and the goodness in all human beings.

In recognition of his contributions, on June 30, 2006, the University of Kansas Medical Center named an Endowed Chair in Orthomolecular Medicine and Research in honor of "Dr. Hugh." The brochure announcing the endowment states, "As a champion and tireless investigator for the use of intravenous vitamin C for cancer, infectious diseases and fibromyalgia, Riordan's seminal work has National Institute of Health (NIH) peer review support for his position on intravenous vitamin C use in cancer cases."

Hugh's death was a major shock. In the weeks and months following his death the work of The Center continued but the staff found it difficult to stay focused. The work went on but it languished. Since Hugh was such a charismatic and compassionate leader, the void he left was difficult to fill.

By 2009 it became evident that changes had to be made and that the staff, loyal as they were, needed to be revitalized. A few staff members were encouraged to resign. With the leadership of Hugh's son Brian (a professional in re-organizing companies), and aided by the expertise of son Neil Riordan (a medical researcher and pioneer in his own right), The Center began a serious self-analysis and renewal process. Changes included additions to the Board of Directors, a new website and the retirement of The Center's name. ***The Center for the Improvement of Human Functioning*** became, simply, ***The Riordan Clinic*** complete with a striking new blue and white logo.

A seed upon rich soil grows. As of this writing the research continues. See the Clinic Website at www.riordanclinic.org for their health related programs and the most recent studies.

Hugh liked "sayings" and had them written on the walls of The Center for inspiration. My favorite saying, and the one that "says it all" regarding Hugh was this, from Benjamin Franklin: "If everyone is thinking alike, then no one is thinking."

Jan Riordan
Wichita, Kansas
November 2011

Favorite Sayings of Hugh D. Riordan

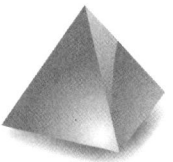

*"Do not follow where the path may lead.
Go instead where there is no path and leave a trail."*
ANONYMOUS

*"While they were saying, it cannot
be done, it was done!"*
ANONYMOUS

*"If everyone is thinking alike,
Then no one is thinking."*
BENJAMIN FRANKLIN

*"Once you know, it is impossible to not know.
And you are forever changed."*
HUGH D. RIORDAN

*"It is impossible for anyone to begin to learn
what he thinks he already knows."*
EPICTETUS

*"We are continually faced
by great opportunities brilliantly disguised as
insolvable problems."*
ANONYMOUS

Journal Articles

Efficacy of oral DMSA and intravenous EDTA in chelation of toxic metals and improvement of the number of stem/ progenitor cells in circulation
Nina Mikirova, Joseph Casciari, Ronald Hunninghake
Translational Biomedicine 2011; 2: 2

Effect of Weight Reduction on Cardiovascular Risk Factors and CD34-positive Cells in Circulation
Nina Mikirova, Joseph Casciari, Ronald Hunninghake, Margaret M Beezley
Int. J. Med. Sci. 2011; 8: 445-452

EDTA Chelation Therapy in the Treatment of Toxic Metals Exposure
Nina Mikirova, Joseph Casciari, Ronald Hunninghake, Neil Riordan
Spatula DD. 2011; 1(2): 81-89

Increased Level of Circulating Endothelial Microparticles and Cardiovascular Risk Factors
Mikirova1 NA, Casciari JJ, Hunninghake RE and Riordan NH
Journal of Clinic & Experimental Cardiology 2011, 2:4 (1 April 2011)

Intravenous ascorbic acid to prevent and treat cancer-associated sepsis?
Ichim TE, Minev B, Braciak T, Luna B, Hunninghake R, Mikirova NA, Jackson JA, Gonzalez MJ, Miranda Massari JR, Alexandrescu DT, Dasanu C, Bogin V, Ancans J, Stevens RBRIAN, Markosian B, Koropatnick J, Chen CS, Riordan NH
Journal of Translational Medicine 2011, 9:25 (4 March 2011)

Vitamin D Concentrations, Endothelial Progenitor Cells, and Cardiovascular Risk Factors
Mikirova NA, Belcaro G, Jackson JA, Riordan NH
Panminerva Medica 2010, 52:(Suppl. 1 to No. 2) (June 2010)

Circulating Endothelial Progenitor Cells and Erectile Dysfunction: Possibility of Nutritional Intervention?
Ichim TE, Zhong Z, Mikirova NA, Jackson JA, Hunninghake R, Mansilla E, Marin G, NúÃ±ez L, Patel AN, Angle N, Murphy MP, Dasanu CA, Alexan-drescu DT, Bogin V, Riordan NH
Panminerva Medica 2010, 52:(Suppl. 1 to No. 1) (June 2010)

Urine Pyrroles and Other Orthomolecular : Tests in Patients With ADD/ADHD
Jackson JA, Braud M, Neathery S
Orthomolecular Medicine, 2010, 25(1):39-41

Mitochondria, Energy and Cancer: The Relationship with Ascorbic Acid
Gonzalez MJ, Rosario-Perez G, Guzman AM, Miranda-Massari JR, Duconge J, Lavergne J, Fernandez N, Ortiz N, Quintero del Rio AI, Mikirova NA, Riordan NH, Ricart CM
Orthomolecular Medicine, 2010, 25(1):29-38

Nutraceutical Augmentation of Circulating Endothelial Progenitor Cells and Hematopoietic Stem Cells in Human Subjects
Mikirova NA, Jackson JA, Hunninghake R, Kenyon J, Chan KWH, Swindlehurst CA, Minev B, Patel A, Murphy MP, Smith L, Ramos F, Alexandrescu D, Ichim TE, Riordan NH
Journal of Translational Medicine 2010, 8:34 (5 Feb 2010)

Ascorbate inhibition of angiogenesis in aortic rings ex vivo and subcutaneous Matrigel plugs in vivo
Mikirova NA, Casciari JJ, Riordan NH
Journal of Angiogenesis Research 2010, 2:2 (18 Jan 2010)

Circulating endothelial progenitor cells: a new approach to anti-aging medicine?
Mikirova NA, Jackson JA, Hunninghake R, Kenyon J, Chan KWH, Swindlehurst CA, Minev B, Patel AN, Murphy MP, Smith L, Alexandrescu DT, Ichim TE, Riordan NH
Journal of Translational Medicine 2009, 7:106 (15 Dec 2009)

Vitamin D (25-OH-D3) Status of 200 Chronically Ill Outpatients Treated at The Center
Jackson JA, Kirby RK, Braud M, Moore K
Orthomolecular Medicine, 2009, 24(2):88-90

Inhibition of Intracranial Glioma Growth by Endometrial Regenerative Cells
Han X, Meng X, Yin Z, Rogers A, Zhong J, Rillema P, Jackson J, Ichim T, Minev B, Carrier E, Patel A, Murphy M, Min W, Riordan N
Cell Cycle, 2009, 8(4):1-5 Feb
Declining Fruit and Vegetable Nutrient Composition: What is the Evidence?
Davis D
HortScience, 2009, 44(1):15-19 Feb

Discerning the Mauve Factor, Part 1
McGinnis W, Audhya T, Walsh W, Jackson J, McLaren-Howard J, Lewis A, Lauda P, Bibus D, Jurnak F, Lietha R, Hoffer A
Alternative Therapies, 2008, 14(2):40-50 *Courtesy of Alternative Therapies in Health and Medicine, © 2008*

Discerning the Mauve Factor, Part 2
McGinnis W, Audhya T, Walsh W, Jackson J, McLaren-Howard J, Lewis A, Lauda P, Bibus D, Jurnak F, Lietha R, Hoffer A
Alternative Therapies, 2008, 14(3):56-62 *Courtesy of Alternative Therapies in Health and Medicine, Â© 2008*

Granulocyte Activity in Patients with Cancer and Healthy Subjects
Mikirova N, Klykov A, Jackson J, Riordan N
Cancer Biology and Therapy, 2008, 7(9):41-46

Anti-angiogenic Effect of High Doses of Ascorbic Acid
Mikirova N, Ichim T, Riordan N
Journal of Translational Medicine, 2008, 6:50

A Child with Metastatic Sarcoma and a Patient with Cancer of the Head of the Pancreas
Jackson J, Hunninghake R, Kirby R, Krier C, Lewis R
Orthomolecular Medicine, 2008, 23(1):41-42

Differential Effect of Alpha-lipoic Acid on Healthy Peripheral Blood Lymphocytes and Leukemic Cells
Mikirova N, Jackson J, Riordan N
Orthomolecular Medicine, 2008, 23(2):83-89

Energy Efficient (toxic?) Light Bulbs
Jackson J, Benson L
Orthomolecular Medicine, 2008, 23(4):182

Pharmacokinetics of Vitamin C: Insights into the Oral and Intravenous Administration of Ascorbate
Duconge J, Miranda-Massari J, Gonzalez M, Jackson J, Warnock W, Riordan N
Puero Rico Health Sciences Journal, 2008, 27(1):7-19

Endometrial Regenerative Cells: A Novel Stem Cell Population
Meng X, Ichim T, Zhong J, Rogers A, Yin Z, Jackson J, Wang H, Ge W, Bogin V, Chan KW, Thebaud B, Riordan NH
Journal of Translational Medicine , 2007, 5:57

Schedule-Dependence in Cancer Therapy: What is the True Scenario for Vitamin C?
Duconge J, Miranda-Massari J, Gonzalez M, Riordan N
Orthomolecular Medicine, 2007, 22(1):21-26

Hidden Food Sensitivities: A Common Cause of Many Illnesses
Jackson J, Neathery S, Kirby R
Orthomolecular Medicine, 2007, 22(1):27-30

PYRAMID ON THE PRAIRIE

A Tired, Achy, Depressed High School Senior
Krier C, Kirby, Jackson J
Orthomolecular Medicine, 2007, 22(2):75-76

The Effect of High Dose IV Vitamin C on Plasma Antioxidant Capacity and Level of Oxidative Stress in Cancer Patients and Healthy Subjects
Mikirova N, Jackson J, Riordan N
Orthomolecular Medicine, 2007, 22(3):153-160

Intravenously Administered Vitamin C as Cancer Therapy Three Cases
Padayatty S, Riordan H, Hewitt S, Katz A, Hoffer L, Levine M
Canadian Medical Association Journal, 2006, 174(7):937-942

Cancer is a Functional Repair Tissue
Meng X, Riordan N
Medical Hypotheses, 2006, 66:486-490

Vitamin C as an Ergogenic Aid
Gonzalez M, Miranda J, Riordan H
Orthomolecular Medicine, 2006, 20(2):100-102

Co-learner/patients comments on treatment
Jackson J, Benson L
Orthomolecular Medicine, 2006, 21(3):157-158

False Positive Finger Stick Blood Glucose Readings After High-Dose Intravenous Vitamin C
Jackson J, Hunninghake R, Krier C, Kirby R, Hyland G
Orthomolecular Medicine, 2006, 21(4):188-190

Tumor Growth Parameters of In-Vivo Human Breast Carcinoma: A Proposed Mathematical Model for Tumor Growth Kinetics
Gonzalez M, Herrera F, Miranda-Massari J, Guzman A, Riordan N, Ricart C
Puero Rico Health Sciences Journal, 2006, 25(1):71-73

Activation of Raf1 and the ERK Pathway in Response to L-ascorbic Acid in Acute Myeloid Leukemia Cells
Park S, Park C, Hahm E, Kim K, Kimler B, Lee S, Park H, Lee S, Kim W, Jung C, Park K, Riordan H, Lee J
Cellular Signalling, 2005, 17:111-119

Trade-Offs in Agriculture and Nutrition
Davis D
Food Technology, 2005, 59(3):120

Journal Articles

Orthomolecular Oncology Review: Ascorbic Acid and Cancer 25 Years Late
Gonzalez M, Miranda-Massari J, Mora E, Guzman A, Riordan N, Riordan H, Casciari J, Jackson J, Roman-Franco A
Integrative Cancer Therapies, 2005, 4(1):32-44

Monitoring of ATP Levels in Red Blood Cells and T Cells of Healthy and Ill Subjects and the Effects of Age on Mitochondrial Potential
Mikirova N, Riordan H, Kirby K, Klykov A, Jackson J
Orthomolecular Medicine, 2005, 20(1):50-58

Payment for Treatment of Symptoms but not for a Cure: One Patient's Experience
Jackson J, Riordan H, McLeod M
Orthomolecular Medicine, 2005, 20(2):111-112

Anemia, Failure to Grow, Ulcerative Colitis and Weight-Loss in a Young Girl
Jackson J, Riordan H, Hunninghake R
Orthomolecular Medicine, 2005, 20(3):191-192

Screening for Vitamin C in the Urine: Is it Clinically Significant?
Jackson J, Wong K, Krier C, Riordan H
Orthomolecular Medicine, 2005, 20(4):259-261

Effects of High Dose Ascorbate Administration on L-10 Tumor Growth in Guinea Pigs
Casciari J, Riordan H, Miranda-Massari J, Gonzalez M
Puero Rico Health Sciences Journal, 2005, 24(2):145-150

A Pilot Clinical Study of Continuous Intravenous Ascorbate in Terminal Cancer Patients
Riordan H, Casciari J, Gonzalez M, Riordan N, Miranda-Massari J, Jackson J
Puero Rico Health Sciences Journal, 2005, 24(4):269-276

Exploring the Parameters of Paramagnetic Forces
Epp M, Riordan H
Acres USA, 2004, 18-21 May

Vitamin C Pharmacokinetics: Implications for Oral and Intravenous Use
Padayatty S, Sun H, Wang Y, Riordan H, Hewitt S, Katz A, Wesley R, Levine M
Annals of Internal Medicine, 2004, 140:533-7

L-Ascorbic Acid Induces Apoptosis in Acute Myeloid Leukemia Cells via Hydrogen Peroxide-Mediated Mechanisms
Park S, Han S, Park C, Hahm E, Lee S, Park H, Lee S, Kim W, Jung C, Park K, Riordan H, Kimler B, Kim K, Lee J
International Journal of Biochemistry & Cell Biology, 2004, 36:2180-95

PYRAMID ON THE PRAIRIE

L-Ascorbic Acid Represses Constitutive Activation of NF-KB and COX-2 Expression in Human Acute Myeloid Leukemia, HL-60
Han S, Kim K, Hahm E, Lee S, Surh Y, Park H, Kim W, Jung C, Lee M, Park K, Yang J, Yoon S, Riordan N, Riordan H, Kimler B, Park C, Lee J, Park S
Journal of Cellular Biochemistry, 2004, 93(2):257-270

Changes in USDA Food Composition Data for 43 Garden Crops, 1950 to 1999
Davis D, Epp M, Riordan H
Journal of the American College of Nutrition, 2004, 23(6):669-682

A Patient Who Said "no" to Surgery, and Was Happy She Did
Jackson J, Riordan H
Orthomolecular Medicine, 2004, 19(1):54-55

Cell Membrane Fatty Acid Composition Differs Between Normal and Malignant Cell Lines
Meng X, Riordan N, Riordan H, Mikirova N, Jackson J, Gonzalez M, Miranda-Massari J, Mora E, Castillo W
Puero Rico Health Sciences Journal, 2004, 23(2):103-106

Erythrocyte Membrane Fatty Acid Composition in Cancer Patients
Mikirova N, Riordan H, Jackson J, Wong K, Miranda-Massari J, Gonzalez M
Puero Rico Health Sciences Journal, 2004, 23(2):107-113

Intravenous Vitamin C as a Chemotherapy Agent: A Report on Clinical Cases
Riordan H, Riordan N, Jackson J, Casciari J, Hunninghake R, Gonzalez M, Mora E, Miranda-Massari J, Rosario N, Rivera A
Puero Rico Health Sciences Journal, 2004, 23(2):115-118

Intravenous Ascorbic Acid as a Treatment for Severe Jellyfish Stings
Kumar S, Miranda-Massari J, Gonzalez M, Riordan H
Puero Rico Health Sciences Journal, 2004, 23(4):125-126

Effect of Vitamin C Supplementation on Ex Vivo Immune Cell Functioning
Casciari J, Riordan H, Mikirova N, Austin J
Orthomolecular Medicine, 2003, 18(2):83-92

Urine Pyrroles in Patients with Cancer
Jackson J, Riordan H, Bramhall N, Neathery S
Orthomolecular Medicine, 2003, 18(1):41-42

Journal Articles

Detection of Energy Metabolism Level in Cancer Patients by Fluorescence Emission from Serum
Mikirova NA, Riordan HD, Rillema P
Orthomolecular Medicine, 2003, 18(1):9-24

Intravenous Ascorbic Acid: Protocol for its Application and Use
Riordan H, Hunninghake R, Riordan N, Jackson J, Meng X, Taylor P, Casciari J, Gonzalez M, Miranda-Massari J, Mora E, Rosario N, Rivera A
Puero Rico Health Sciences Journal, 2003, 22(3):287-290

Preventive Health Screening Program in an Industrial Setting: Identifying Health Risks and Nutritional Deficiencies
Jackson J, Riordan H, Tiemeyer J, Revard C, Neathery S
Orthomolecular Medicine, 2002, 17(1):49-52

Sixteen-Year History with High Dose Intravenous Vitamin C Treatment for Various Types of Cancer and Other Diseases
Jackson J, Riordan H, Bramhall N, Neathery S
Orthomolecular Medicine, 2002, 17(2):117-119

Assessment of Granulocyte Activity with Application to Healthy and Ill Subjects
Mikirova N, Riordan H, Klykov A
Orthomolecular Medicine, 2002, 17(3):151-161

Vitamin C and Oxidative DNA Damage Revisited
Gonzalez M, Riordan H, Miranda-Massari J
Orthomolecular Medicine, 2002, 17(4):225-228

Detection of the Level of Energy Metabolism in Patients with Chronic Fatigue Syndrome by Fluorescence Emission from Serum
Mikirova NA, Riordan HD, Rillema P
Orthomolecular Medicine, 2002, 17(4):197-208

Inhibition of Human Breast Carcinoma Cell Proliferation by Ascorbate and Copper
Gonzalez M, Mora E, Miranda-Massari J, Matta E, Riordan H, Riordan N
Puero Rico Health Sciences Journal, 2002, 21(1):21-23

Orthomolecular Oncology: A Mechanistic View of Antravenous Ascorbate's Chemotherapeutic Activity
Gonzalez M, Miranda-Massari J, Mora E, Jimenez I, Matos M, Riordan H, Casciari J, Riordan N, Rodriguez M, Guzman A
Puero Rico Health Sciences Journal, 2002, 21(1):39-41

Effects of a High Molecular Mass Convolvulus Arvensis Extract on Tumor Growth and Angiogenesis
Meng X, Riordan N, Casciari J, Zhu Y, Zhong J, Gonzalez M, Miranda-Massari J, Riordan H
Puero Rico Health Sciences Journal, 2002, 21(4):323-328

Cytotoxicity of Ascorbate, Lipoic Acid, and Other Antioxidants in Hollow Fibre in Vitro Tumours
Casciari J, Riordan N, Schmidt T, Meng X, Jackson J, Riordan H
British Journal of Cancer, 2001, 84(11):1544-1550

Urine Pyrroles Revisited
Jackson J, Riordan H, Neathery S, Mayer K
Orthomolecular Medicine, 2001, 16(1):47-48

The Effect of Alternating Magnetic Field Exposure and Vitamin C on Cancer Cells
Mikirova N, Jackson J, Casciari, Riordan H
Orthomolecular Medicine, 2001, 16(3):177-182

Three Patients, Three Medical Conditions, Three Successful Outcomes
Jackson J, Riordan H, Hunninghake R, Lewis R
Orthomolecular Medicine, 2001, 16(4):238-240

Urine Indican as an Indicator of Disease
Jackson J, Riordan H, Neathery S
Orthomolecular Medicine, 2000, 15(1):18-20

Lycopene: Its Role in Health and Disease
Jackson J, Riordan H, Revard C, Tiemeyer J
Orthomolecular Medicine, 2000, 15(2):103-104

Comparison of Hair Copper, Zinc, Aluminum and Lead in Patients with Elevated and Normal Urine Pyrrole Levels
Jackson J, Riordan H, Neathery S, Tiemeyer J
Orthomolecular Medicine, 2000, 15(3):139-140

Clinical and Experimental Experiences with Intravenous Vitamin C
Riordan N, Casciari J, Riordan H
Orthomolecular Medicine, 2000, 15(4):201-213

Different Fatty Acid Composition Between Normal and Malignant Cell Lines
Meng X, Riordan N, Riordan H, Jackson J, Zhong J, Li Y, Gonzalez M, McClune B, Pappan K
BioMedicina, 1999, 2(4):s5-s7 May

Journal Articles

Intravenous EDTA Chelation Treatment of a Patient with Atherosclerosis
Jackson J, Riordan H, Schultz M, Lewis R
Orthomolecular Medicine, 1999, 14(2):91-92

Headache: A Common Complaint with Complicated Causes
Jackson J, Riordan H, Hunninghake R, Revard C
Orthomolecular Medicine, 1999, 14(3):169-171

Candida Albicans: The Hidden Infection
Jackson J, Riordan H, Hunninghake R, Mayer K
Orthomolecular Medicine, 1999, 14(4):198-200

Antioxidants as Chemopreventive Agents for Breast Cancer
Gonzalez M, Riordan N, Riordan H
BioMedicina, 1998, 1(4):120-127 April

Rethinking Vitamin C and Cancer: An Update on Nutritional Oncology
Gonzalez M, Mora E, Riordan N, Riordan H, Mojica P
Cancer Prevention International, 1998, 3:215-224

The Nutrition Evaluation Questionnaire as a Diagnostic Aid
Jackson J, Riordan H, Fougeron K, Hunninghake R
Orthomolecular Medicine, 1998, 13(1):28-30

High-Dose Intravenous Vitamin C in the Treatment of a Patient with Renal Cell Carcinoma of the Kidney
Riordan H, Jackson J, Riordan N, Schultz M
Orthomolecular Medicine, 1998, 13(2):72-73

Joint and Muscle Pain, Various Arthritic Conditions and Food Sensitivities
Jackson J, Riordan H, Hunninghake R, Neathery S
Orthomolecular Medicine, 1998, 13(3):168-172

Histamine Levels in Health and Disease
Jackson J, Riordan H, Neathery S, Revard C
Orthomolecular Medicine, 1998, 13(4):236-240

Pilot Study of the Effects of Thymus Protein on Elevated Epstein-Barr Virus Titers
Riordan N, Jackson J, Riordan H
Townsend Letter for Doctors & Patients, 1998, 78-79 Feb/Mar

Red Blood Cell Fatty Acids as a Diagnostic Tool
Jackson J, Riordan H, Riordan N, Neathery S
Orthomolecular Medicine, 1997, 12(1):20-22

Urinary Pyrrole in Health and Disease
Jackson J, Riordan H, Neathery S, Revard C
Orthomolecular Medicine, 1997, 12(2):96-98

Ascorbic Acid Effect on Plasma Amino Acids
Jackson J, Riordan H, Neathery S, Riordan N
Orthomolecular Medicine, 1997, 12(3):164-165

The Patient With a Harmful Hobby and the the Depressed Teen-Age Patient
Jackson J, Riordan H, Hunninghake R
Orthomolecular Medicine, 1997, 12(4):219-220

Antioxidants and Pro-Oxidants: A Commentary About Their Appent Discrepant Role in Carcinogenesis
Gonzalez M, Lopez D, Argulies M, Riordan N
Age, 1996, 19:17-18

The Paradoxical Role of Lipid Peroxidation on Carcinogenesis and Tumor Growth: A Commentary
Gonzalez M, Riordan N
Medical Hypotheses, 1996, 46(6):503-504

Coronary Artery Occlusion, Chelation and Cholesterol in a 49-Year Old Pilot
Jackson J, Hunninghake R, Riordan H, Sarwar Y
Orthomolecular Medicine, 1996, 11(1):14

Intravenous Vitamin C in a Terminal Cancer Patient
Riordan N, Jackson J, Riordan H
Orthomolecular Medicine, 1996, 11(2):80-82

Trials and Tribulations of a Three-Year Old
Jackson J, Riordan H, Doran L, Hunninghake R
Orthomolecular Medicine, 1996, 11(3):145-146

Epstein-Barr Virus Infections in Patients
Jackson J, Riordan H, Hunninghake R, Meng X, Sarwar Y
Orthomolecular Medicine, 1996, 11(4):208-210

Intravenous Ascorbate as a Tumor Cytotoxic Chemotherapeutic Agent
Riordan N, Riordan H, Meng X, Li Y, Jackson J
Medical Hypotheses, 1995, 44(3):207-213

Journal Articles

The Cytotoxic Food Sensitivity Test: An Important Diagnostic Tool
Jackson J, Riordan H, Neathery S, Guinn C
Orthomolecular Medicine, 1995, 10(1):60-61

High Dose Intravenous Vitamin C and Long Time Survival of a Patient with Cancer of Head of the Pancreas
Jackson J, Riordan H, Hunninghake R, Riordan N
Orthomolecular Medicine, 1995, 10(2):87-88

Agitation, Allergies and Attention Deficit Disorder in an 11-Year Old Boy
Jackson J, Hunninghake R, Riordan H, Doran L
Orthomolecular Medicine, 1995, 10(4):130

Improved Microplate Fluorometer Counting of Viable Tumor and Normal Cells
Riordan H, Riordan N, Meng X, Zhong J, Jackson J
Anticancer Research, 1994, 14:927-931

An Unusual Intestinal Parasitic Infection
Yiming L, Jackson J, Riordan N, Riordan H
Orthomolecular Medicine, 1994, 9(1):38

Rheumatoid Arthritis in a Young Male
Riordan H, Jackson J, Hunninghake R
Orthomolecular Medicine, 1994, 9(2):109-110

Auricular Therapy: Diagnosis and Treatment
Jackson J, McCray M, Riordan H, Hunninghake R
Orthomolecular Medicine, 1994, 9(3):157-158

Hyperbaric Oxygen Treatment
Jackson J, Riordan H, Doran L, Riordan N
Orthomolecular Medicine, 1994, 9(4):222-224

Ankylosing Spondylitis
Jackson J, Hunninghake R, Riordan H
Orthomolecular Medicine, 1993, 8(1):51-52

Chronic Abdominal Pain
Jackson J, Hunninghake R, Riordan HN
Orthomolecular Medicine, 1993, 8(2):98

Sarcoidosis
Jackson J, Hunninghake R, Riordan H
Orthomolecular Medicine, 1993, 8(3):136

Beat the Odds
Riordan H, Jackson J, Hunninghake R
Orthomolecular Medicine, 1993, 8(4):227-228

Correlations Between Chronological and Biological Age Levels of Blood Lipids
Tinterrow M, Riordan H, Jackson J, Dirks M
Townsend Letter for Doctors & Patients, 1993, 242-244 Feb/Mar

Improvement of Essential Hypertension After EDTA Intraveneous Infusion
Jackson J, Riordan H
Orthomolecular Medicine, 1992, 7(1):16

Chronic Fatigue and Depression
Riordan H, Jackson J
Orthomolecular Medicine, 1992, 7(2):111-112

Migraine Headaches and Food Sensitivities in a Child
Jackson J, Riordan H, Hunninghake R
Orthomolecular Medicine, 1992, 7(3):146

Illness and Intestinal Parasites
Jackson J, Hunninghake R, Riordan N
Orthomolecular Medicine, 1992, 7(4):202

Some Puzzlements in Life Science Research Methodology
Riordan H
American Clinical Laboratory, 1991, Sept

Topical Ascorbate Stops Prolonged Bleeding from Tooth Extraction
Riordan H, Jackson J
Orthomolecular Medicine, 1991, 6(3&4):202

Recareering Instead of Retiring
Tinterrow M
Phi Delta Epsilon News and Scientific Journal, 1991, 83(2):10-12

Vitamin, Blood Lead, and Urine Pyrrole Levels in Down Syndrome
Jackson J, Riordan H, Neathery S
American Clinical Laboratory, 1990, 8-9 Jan/Feb

Mineral Excretion Associated with EDTA Chelation Therapy
Riordan H, Cheraskin E, Dirks M
Journal of Advancement in Medicine, 1990, 3(2):111-123

Journal Articles

Intravenous EDTA Infusion and the Hemogram
Riordan H, Cheraskin E, Dirks M, Tinterrow M
Journal of Advancement in Medicine, 1990, 3(3):185-188

Case Study: High Dose Intravenous Vitamin C in the Treatment of a Patient with Adrenocarcinoma of the Kidney
Riordan H, Jackson J, Schultz
Orthomolecular Medicine, 1990, 5(1):5-7

Aluminum from a Coffee Pot
Jackson J, Riordan H, Poling C
Lancet, 1989, 333(8641):781-782 Apr

EDTA Chelation/Hypertension Study: Clinical Patterns as Judged by the Cornell Medical Index Questionnaire
Riordan H, Cheraskin E, Dirks M, Tadayon F, Schultz M, Brizendine P
Orthomolecular Medicine, 1989, 4(2):91-95

The Effects of Intravenous EDTA Infusion on the Multichemical Profile
Riordan H, Cheraskin E, Dirks M, Schultz M, Brizendine P
American Clinical Laboratory, 1988, Oct

Electrocardiographic Changes Associated with EDTA Chelation Therapy
Riordan H, Jackson J, Cheraskin E, Dirks M
Journal of Advancement in Medicine, 1988, 1(4):191-194

Another Look at Renal Function and the EDTA Treatment Process
Riordan H, Cheraskin E, Dirks M, Schultz M, Brizendine P
Orthomolecular Medicine, 1987, 2(3):185-187

Behavior and Brain Neurotransmitters: Correlations in Different Strains of Mice
Krehbiel D, Bartel B, Dirks M, Wiens W
Behavioral and Neural Biology, 1986, 46(1):30-45

Changes in Social Behavior and Brain Catecholamines During the Development of Ascorbate Deficiency in Guinea Pigs
Kaufmann P, Wiens W, Dirks M, Krehbiel D
Behavioural Processes, 1986, 13(1-2):13-28

Modulation of Reproductive Output in Drosophila by Spectral Properties of Ambient Light
Bruce B, Wayne W, Marvin D, Hugh R
Canadian Journal of Zoology, 1986, 64(2):537-542

Differences in Human Serum Copper and Zinc Levels in Healthy and Patient Populations
Cheraskin E, Carpenter J, Riordan H
Medical Hypotheses, 1986, 20(1):79-85

Clinical Correlations Between Serum Glucose Variance and Reported Symptoms in Human Subjects
Riordan H, Hinshaw C, Carpenter, Landreth M, Cheraskin E
Medical Hypotheses, 1984, 15(1):67-79

Blood Histamine Level as a Factor in Skin Conductance and Response
Dirks M, Riordan H, Canfield M
Biofeedback and Self Regulation, 1978, 3(2) Jun

A Humanistic Approach to Medical Practic
Riordan H
Dialogue, 1976, 3(4):6-8

About the Author

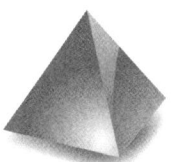

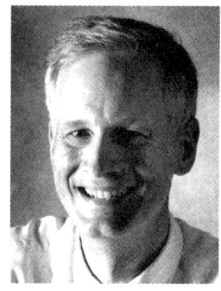

Craig Miner was the Willard W. Garvey Distinguished Professor of Business History at Wichita State University at the time of his death in 2010 at the age of 65. Having earned his undergraduate and master's degrees from WSU, he completed his doctorate in history at the University of Colorado and joined the Wichita State faculty in 1969. Regarded as the foremost historian of Wichita and Kansas history, he taught courses in a variety of topics of US history and economic history as well as advanced research and writing. Dr. Miner served as chair of the history department from 1998-2004 and director of the public history program from 1998-1999. He was the author of 40 books. A past president of the Wichita's Historic Landmark Committee and the Kansas State Historical Society, he also served on the University Press of Kansas Editorial Board and the Board of the Kansas Humanities Council. A wide array of subjects kept Dr. Miner's interest. He learned Egyptian hieroglyphics, Latin, and ancient Greek and enjoyed amateur astronomy, cross-county bicycling, classical guitar, book collecting, and classic cars. He and his wife Susan were devoted to the preservation of their historic landmark home, Hillside Cottage, where they raised their two sons: Hal, who lives with his wife Gretchen in Portland, Oregon, and Wilson, who with his wife Laura resides in San Francisco.

Check out the Wikipedia page for Hugh D. Riordan:
www.wikipedia.org/wiki/Hugh_D_Riordan